Bre

Step by Step
Breast Ultrasound

Rahul Sachdev
MBBS DMRD FICMU
Consultant Radiologist

Manjula Handa Virmani
MBBS MD
Diplomat American Board Radiology
Fellowship Breast Imaging (USA)
Consultant Radiologist

Ashok Khurana
MBBS MD
Consultant Radiologist

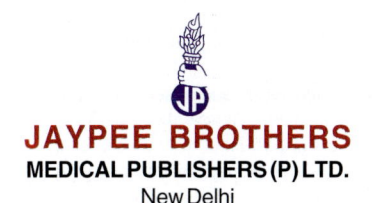

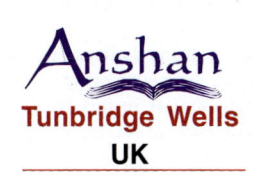

JAYPEE BROTHERS
MEDICAL PUBLISHERS (P) LTD.
New Delhi

Anshan
Tunbridge Wells
UK

First published in the UK by

Anshan Ltd
in 2006
6 Newlands Road
Tunbridge Wells
Kent TN4 9AT, UK

Tel/Fax: +44 (0)1892 557767
E-mail: info@anshan.co.uk
www.anshan.co.uk

Copyright © 2006 by (author)

The right of authors to be identified as the author of this work has been asserted in accordance with the Copyright, Designs and Patents act 1988.

ISBN-10 1 904798 799
ISBN-13 978 1 904798 79 8

British Library Cataloguing in Publication Data
A catalogue record for this book is available from the British Library

All rights reserved. No part of this publication may be reproduced, stored in a retrieval system, or transmitted in any form or by any means, electronic, mechanical, photocopying, recording and/or otherwise without the prior written permission of the publishers. This book may not be lent, resold, hired out or otherwise disposed of by way of trade in any form, binding or cover other than that in which it is published, without the prior consent of the publishers.

Printed in India by Paras Offset Pvt. Ltd., Naraina, New Delhi.

Many of the designations used by manufacturers and sellers to distinguish their products are claimed as trademarks. Where those designations appear in this book and where the publisher was aware of a trademark claim, the designations have been printed in initial capital letters.

PREFACE

Breast Ultrasound has advanced enormously in the last five years, both in quantity and quality. US is used as a primary imaging for under 35's. US is used as second imaging to further characterize all mammographic lesions and in patients with clinical abnormalities not seen on Mammography. US visible lesions are biopsied under US guidance; this enables complex problems to be sorted out.

This book has been designed as a comprehensive work for all health care professionals dealing with breast imaging. It has been divided into 4 Sections to facilitate reading and review. Section 1 is a brief introduction to Breast Ultrasound; Section 2 deals with technical aspects; section 3 contains chapters on benign and malignant lesions; finally Section 4 deals with breast implants.

This book shows some of the pits we have fallen into the last five years, with hints on trying to stay out of them.

Rahul Sachdev
Manjula Handa Virmani
Ashok Khurana

CONTENTS

Section 1: Introduction

1. History of Breast Ultrasound 3

Section 2: Performing Breast Ultrasound

2. Equipment Considerations 9
3. Recent Technical Developments 19
4. Anatomical Considerations 33
5. Patient Positioning 45
6. Scanning Techniques 51
7. Annotating Lesion Location 55
8. Echogenecity 59
9. Reporting and Communication 65
10. Interventional Procedures 71

Section 3: Benign and Malignant Lesions

11. Development and Involution 79
12. Evaluation of a Nipple Discharge 85
13. Assessing the Breast Lump 91
14. Solid Lesions: Benign Versus Malignant 95
15. Solid Lesions: Specific Benign Diagnoses ... 115
16. High Risk and Premalignant Diagnoses 131
17. Cystic Lesions 139

18. **Complex Cystic Lesions** 145
19. **The Male Breast** 161

Section 4: Post-treatment Evaluation

20. **The Augmented Breast** 165
    Index *169*

Section 1

Introduction

Chapter 1

History of Breast Ultrasound

STEP BY STEP BREAST ULTRASOUND

Breast ultrasound (BUS) has come a long way since Wild and Reid in 1951 first imaged a 3 mm mass in the breast using an A mode transducer. Since it did not use ionising radiation, the thrust of BUS in its initial development, was to use it as a possible alternative to conventional X-Ray mammography, as a breast cancer screening tool. Manufacturers directed research towards the development of automated whole breast scanning devices which, however, fell pathetically short of the accuracy offered by conventional mammography. This failure arose from the fact that ultrasound shows poor sensitivity for calcification which is the essential feature to identify in breast screening programmes. It was apparent from these initial experiences nevertheless, that ultrasound offered a unique technique to demonstrate textural details of the normal and abnormal breast in a far superior way to mammography. Whereas both BUS and mammography can identify air, fat, water and calcium, only BUS can differentiate between different water densities. Based on this property, the technique as it is employed today, has emerged as an invaluable adjunct to clinical examination and mammography.

The main classes of *indications* for BUS include:
- Identification and characterisation of palpable and mammographic abnormalities
- Guidance for interventional procedures
- Evaluation of implants
- Screening examinations.

HISTORY OF BREAST ULTRASOUND

The *principal aim* of currently employed Breast Ultrasound techniques is to make a more *specific diagnosis* in patients with *clinical* or *mammographic* findings. As a consequence there has been an appreciable increase in the diagnostic confidence in labelling a lesion as benign and avoiding a biopsy. Equally interestingly, there has also been an increase in the suspicion of malignancy in a small number of lesions, thereby dictating the need for a guided sampling in this subgroup. Population screening for breast cancer detection and microcalcification has not yet met standards of sensitivity for approval by agencies such as the FDA of the United States of America and recent advances in technique and technology are constantly under surveillance for possible approval.

The aims of the examination include:
- Reducing the number of negative biopsies
- Reducing the number of short-interval follow-ups
- Interventional procedure guidance
- To identify and better classify malignant lesions
- Determining extent of malignant disease
- Improving mammographic interpretation
- Improving clinical examination skills.

This handbook attempts to chart out the methods by which BUS can be used efficiently to not only differentiate clinical or mammographic masses as solid versus cystic but to further characterise them to a near close histopathologic diagnosis.

Section 2

Performing Breast Ultrasound

Chapter 2

Equipment Considerations

Technical specifications are a very important prerequisite for good quality breast ultrasound. It is necessary to use equipment that offers very high resolution in the near field close to the skin.

TRANSDUCER FREQUENCY AND STAND-OFFS

The American College of Radiology and the American Institute of Ultrasound in Medicine place a *minimum requirement* of a broadband electronically focused, linear array transducer with a nominal central frequency of 7 MHz or higher. A short axis elevation plane focal length close to the skin is also required. Widely available linear or curved array transducers with 5 MHz frequency are too deeply focused to be of use in optimal visualisation of the breast (Fig. 2.1). These may, however, be useful

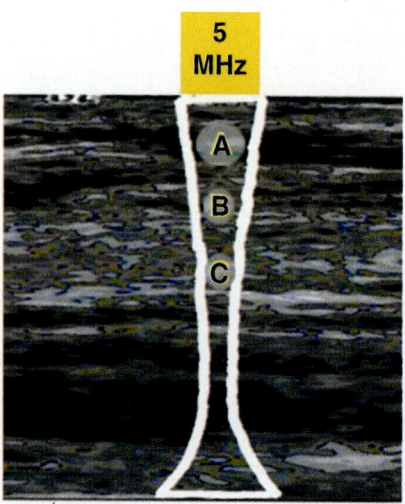

Fig. 2.1: Most 5 MHz transducers are designed for peripheral vascular ultrasound. These are focused at a depth of 30-40 mm. They are, therefore, inadequate for breast ultrasound. Lesion A is superficial and will be subject to volume averaging and therefore either lost to being picked up. A cystic lesion in this location will appear falsely solid. Lesion B will have the same fate. Only lesion C located near the chest wall will be adequately imaged

EQUIPMENT CONSIDERATIONS 11

in thicker and pendulous breasts, in the lactating or inflamed breast and in large implants. Near focussed 7 MHz transducers may also, on occasion, not be optimal for very superficial lesions particularly those in the superficial 6-7 mm depth. This is because of reverberation artefacts, side-lobe artefacts and very small size (Fig. 2.2). In such situations a very thick layer

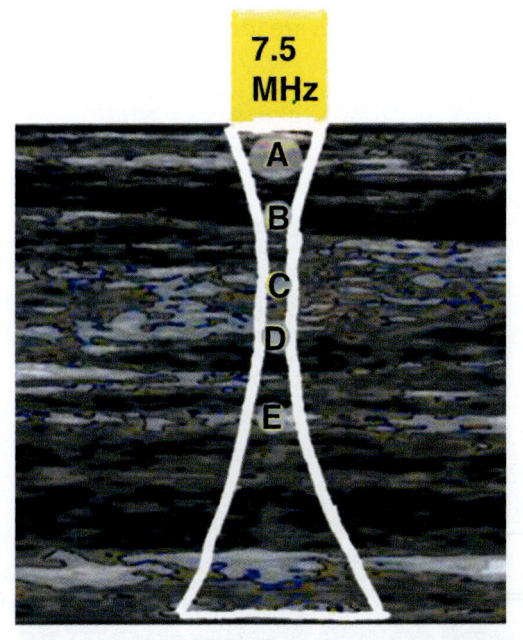

Fig. 2.2: High resolution 7.5-12 MHz transducers show reasonably good focusing through most of the depth of the average breast. Lesions B, C and D would, therefore, be adequately delineated. In the very near field, however, particularly upto 7-8 mm in depth, a lesion (A) can still be missed. Near the chest wall the beam is no longer focused and a lesion (E) may be missed

of jelly or a stand-off pad may be of use (Fig. 2.3). The advantage of a thick layer of jelly compared to a stand-off pad include ease of application, ease of thickness adjustment and the possibility of palpating a lesion at the same time as performing the scan. Stand-off pads offer the advantage of a complete absence of air-bubbles. Conventional stand-off pads of 20-30 mm thickness are not suitable and special stand-off pads of about 7 mm are ideal for breast ultrasound.

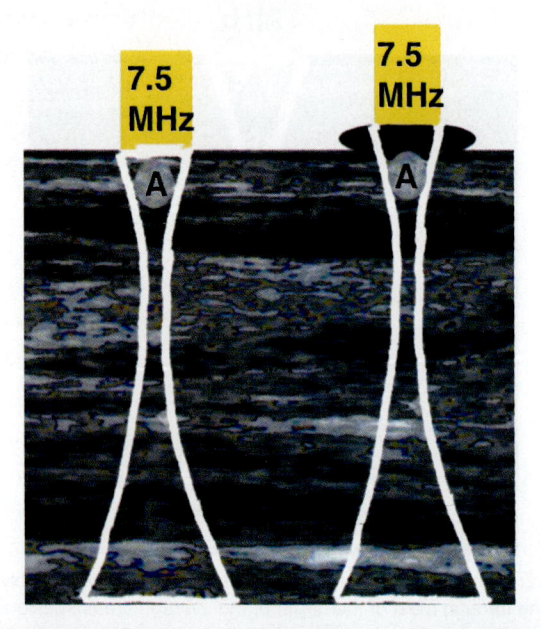

Fig. 2.3: Very near field lesions that are volume averaged and therefore missed using even high frequency transducers can be picked up by using thin stand-off pads or a blob of gel. This brings the first 10 mm of breast tissue within the focal zone of most 7.5-10 MHz transducers

EQUIPMENT CONSIDERATIONS

Resolution

Transducers must offer good spatial and contrast resolution.

Spatial Resolution

Spatial resolution refers to the ability of a system to distinguish between two adjacent points. The lesser the distance between two such points, the better the resolution. Spatial resolution involves *lateral resolution* and *axial resolution*. Lateral resolution refers to distinguishing two points in the *same depth plane* and axial resolution refers to two points in the *same axis* but at different depths. Spatial resolution, thus, involves *three axes* (depth, long axis of the transducer and short axis of the transducer) and *two planes* (lateral and axial). Good lateral resolution at all depths within the breast is necessary to prevent *volume averaging* of pathologic lesions with adjacent normal breast tissue. As a result of *volume averaging*, small lesions may be obscured completely (Fig. 2.4) and cystic areas may appear solid.

The long axis of the linear probe can be *electronically focused*. Continuous electronic focusing may be done on *receive* or *transmit* phases. The degree of electronic focusing on receive depends upon many factors, including number of channels, aperture size, number of elements and number of scan lines. Electronic focusing on transmit depends on many of the same factors as receive focusing, but is more limited. It

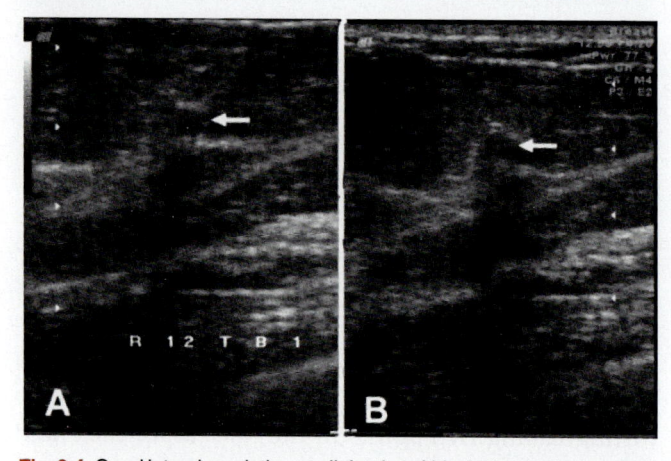

Fig. 2.4: Good lateral resolution at all depths within the breast is necessary to prevent volume averaging of pathologic lesions with adjacent normal breast tissue. As a result of volume averaging, small lesions may be obscured completely. With a 5 MHz transducer this hypoechoic lesion with adjacent calcification is almost missed completely (A), Using a 7.5 MHz transducer gives better delineation of the lesion and its components (B)

depends upon the number of transmit zones. In general, the more transmit zones, the better the lateral resolution. However, increasing the number of transmit zones, decreases the frame rate. Newer equipment offers more than four transmit focal zones and still maintains an acceptable frame rate of 12 frames per second. In general, multiple transmit focal zones in the first 20 mm are very beneficial in breast ultrasound.

The elevation plane (short axis) of the probe in the commonly available 1-D probes cannot be electronically focused because these are only one element wide. The elevation plane is focused at a fixed depth by an *acoustic lens*. The depth is decided by the designer and manufacturer. In order to use the same transducer for peripheral vascular applications and varied small parts applications, some manufacturers use a deeper focal plane even with 7 MHz transducers. These are not optimal for imaging the breast. With 1.5-D and multidimensional probes, focusing can be achieved electronically and with lenses of different shapes (Fig. 2.5). Dedicated small parts or near field probes for breast ultrasound should be focused at about 15 mm or even more superficially. Recently available, relatively lower end equipment that uses *multiplexing algorithms*

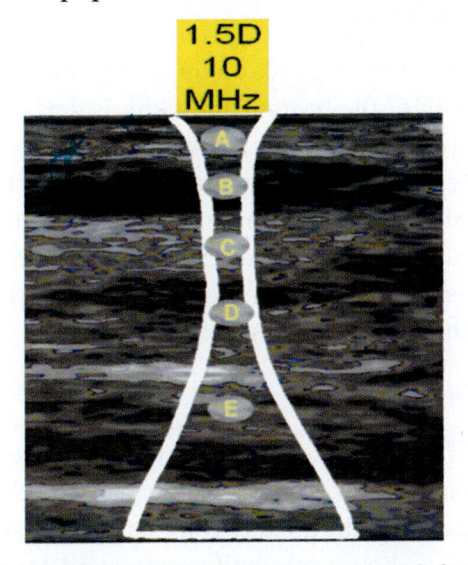

Fig. 2.5: 1.5 and Multidimensional probes use electronic focusing and multiple lenses as well. This greatly improves near field resolution (A) and resolution through most of the breast tissue (B to D). Lesions near the chest wall (E) may, however, still be missed

with fewer hardware channels is offering challenges to high resolution systems with numerous hardware channels. 5MHz linear array probes are usually designed in the larger perspective of use in peripheral vascular applications and are focused in the elevation plane of about 30 to 40 mm. This is too deep for most breast imaging since the elevation plane would be focused in the pectoralis muscle in most patients. In general a 7.5 to 13 MHz transducer, with an elevation plane of about 15 mm, is the best breast ultrasound transducer currently available.

Axial Resolution

Axial resolution depends on transducer frequency and bandwidth of the beam. Bandwidth is determined by transducer material and pulse length. The higher the frequency, the shorter the wavelength and the better the axial resolution. Similarly, the shorter the pulse length, the better the axial resolution. Axial resolution is necessary to delineate the mammary ducts and to define the pseudocapsule of benign lesions.

Contrast Resolution

Contrast resolution is important to make breast lesions more conspicuous and thereby increase the chances of being spotted. Additionally, contrast resolution permits distinctions between small subtle solid lesions and surrounding fatty or glandular tissue. The higher the

EQUIPMENT CONSIDERATIONS

contrast resolution, the higher the clutter, reverberations and sidelobe artefacts. Industrially, therefore, there is a trade-off between higher frequencies and broad bandwidth on the one hand and a reduced contrast resolution on the other.

Chapter 3

Recent Technical Developments

Technology changes everyday and at a very rapid pace. Breast ultrasound is no exception. Most manufacturers have added numerous software and hardware manipulations to enhance the yield of a breast ultrasound examination. This chapter dwells on these recent and not so recent additions to the basic Real Time 2D grey scale, high frequency, broad-bandwidth, high dynamic range setting, breast ultrasound examination.

HARMONIC IMAGING

Lower frequency elements of the ultrasound beam generate side lobes and backscatter which reduce contrast resolution. By receiving only higher frequency components, much of the artefact is excluded from the image and only true information is preserved. This is possible by using harmonic imaging. In this technique, the beam is transmitted at one frequency and received at multiples of the transmitted frequency. In breast ultrasound the *first harmonic*, which is received at twice the transmitted frequency is used.

Harmonic imaging can be achieved by *simple filtration* of the returning beam. This would, however, reduce penetration into the deeper layers. Also, this would result in a narrow bandwidth which reduces axial resolution. A reduced axial resolution diminishes the visualisation of duct walls and pseudocapsules, which is so useful in differentiating benign from malignant disease. A high technology alternative to

RECENT TECHNICAL DEVELOPMENTS

simple filtration is *digital encoding* of the beam. This improves penetration with higher frequencies and permits receiving the doubled frequency of the returning echoes as a broad bandwidth. Reverberations, side lobes, cluster and speckle are all reduced.

This offers the following advantages:
- Indeterminate lesions with doubtful internal echoes are revealed as being truly cystic (Fig. 3.1)
- Cysts that become more echogenic with harmonics are truly echogenic
- Near field reverberation is reduced, thereby improving visualisation of extravasated implant gel between the fibrous capsule and the implant shell

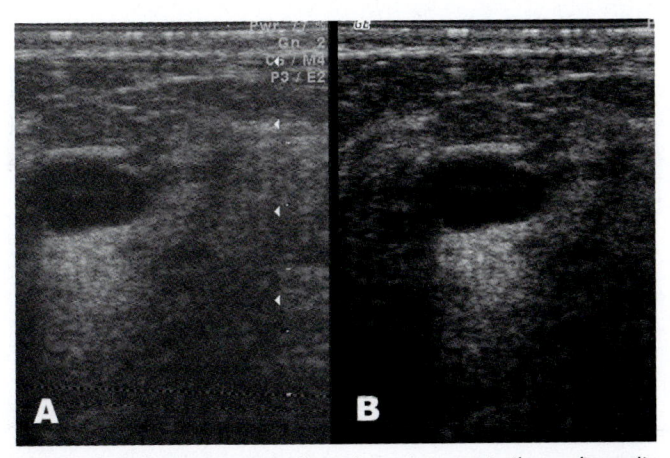

Fig. 3.1: Digital encoding of the beam improves penetration and permits receiving the first harmonic as a broad bandwidth. Doubtfully hypoechoic lesions can therefore be more convincingly assessed as being truly cystic

- Solid nodules appear more hypoechoic (Fig. 3.2) and are, therefore, less likely to be missed
- The pseudocapsule of benign lesions is better defined (Fig. 3.3)
- Implant shells are more clearly contoured
- Speckle is markedly reduced, thereby enhancing the visualisation of calcification (Fig. 3.4).

The limitations of harmonic imaging are minor and include:
- Decreased far field penetration in a small number of cases
- Reduced frame rate
- Restricted benefit in the very-near near field.

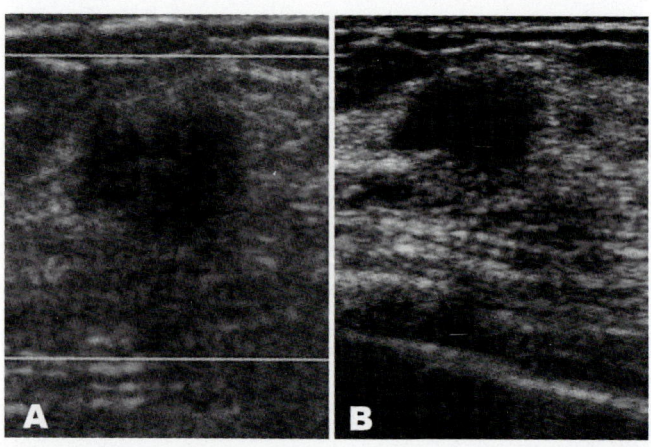

Fig. 3.2: When harmonic imaging is used, a solid nodule (A) appears less solid and more hypoechoic (B). These lesions are, therefore, less likely to be missed

RECENT TECHNICAL DEVELOPMENTS 23

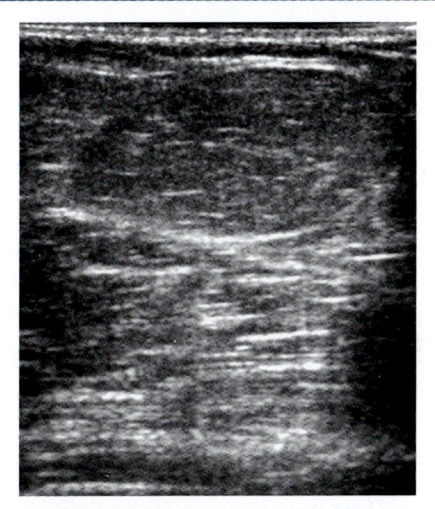

Fig. 3.3: A thin echogenic capsule is a reliable sign of a benign lesion. Harmonic imaging enhances the demonstration of this sign

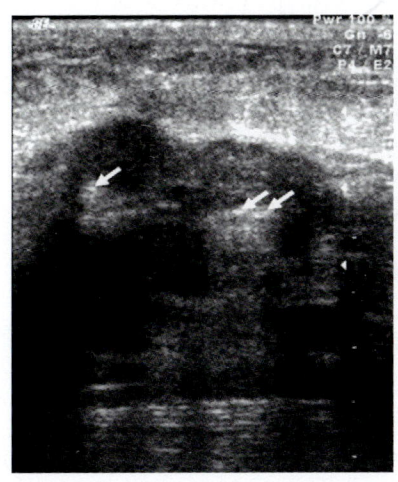

Fig. 3.4: It is conventionally believed that calcification cannot be picked up by ultrasound. With newer equipment this is not true any more. Calcification is being increasingly picked up especially when harmonic imaging is used. The sensitivity of ultrasound still does not match the sensitivity of mammography for calcification. On ultrasound most calcific foci are volume averaged and do not cast a distal acoustic shadow. This illustration shows multiple foci of calcification in a malignant lesion arising in a fibroadenoma

AUTOMATED TISSUE OPTIMISATION

Photoediting software uses a post-processing function on single freeze frame digital images whereby the gray-scale is remapped over the range of gray shades actually present in an image to reduce the haze in the image because of high dynamic range settings. Some manufacturers have incorporated this technology into real time ultrasound of the breast and call it Automatic Tissue Optimisation (ATO). Using the technique improves contrast resolution.

SPATIAL COMPOUNDING

With this technique, images are constructed from variably *multiple sweeps* by *beam steering*. This is a real time procedure which builds up real echoes and averages out artefacts to reveal temporally and spatially compounded images as long as the transducer position is constant. The technique uses an inherently low frame rate which exaggerates motion artefact and is marked by *high persistence*. This is overcome by doing a complete survey using lower sweep numbers and following this up with a targeted evaluation with higher sweep numbers.

Advantages include:
- Better visualisation of the pseudocapsule of benign lesions
- Enhanced delineation of Cooper's ligaments
- Improved delineation of malignant spiculation (Fig. 3.5).

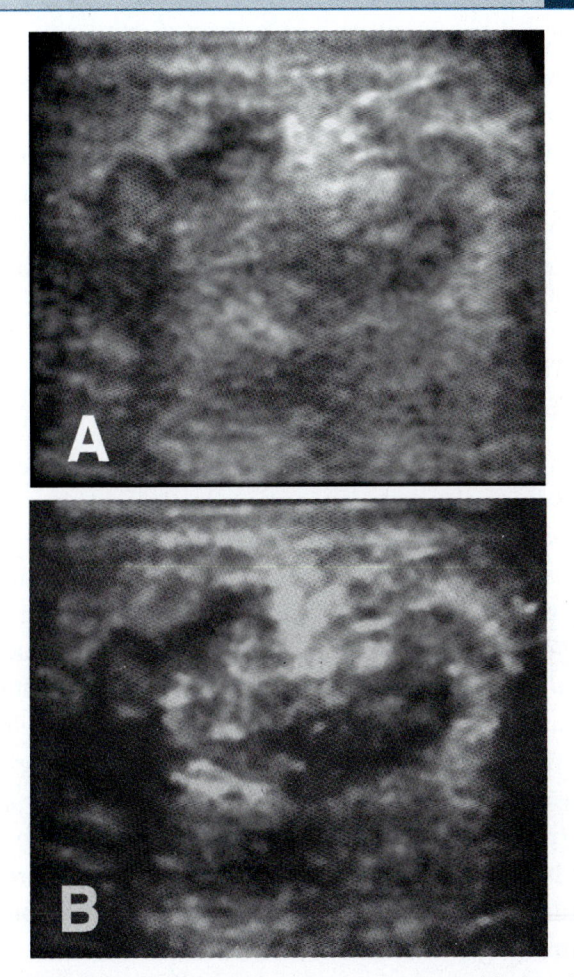

Fig. 3.5: Spatially compounded images are constructed from multiple sweeps using electronic beam steering. This excludes artifacts and the high persistence enhances edge delineation. When hypoechoic lesions which are poorly delineated from surrounding normal breast tissues (A) are spatially compounded, spiculated margins (B) become more distinctive, thereby enhancing the suspicion of malignancy

Limitations include:
- Decreased enhanced through transmission in larger cysts
- Absent distal acoustic enhancement in smaller cysts
- Reduced distal acoustic shadowing in desmoplastic carcinomas.

Coded harmonics and spatial compounding may be used together but are marked by a very low frame rate.

VIRTUAL CONVEX IMAGING AND EXTENDED FIELD OF VIEW

50 mm long transducers with a larger number of transducer elements, no increase in element size, and, increased effective number of channels are becoming available. The central portion functions as a linear array and the periphery as a phased array to give a virtual convex large field of view. These are useful to enhance *global visualisation* and reveal the *relationships* of multiple lesions (Figs 3.6 to 3.8) in the same breast as well as relationship with ducts. Extended field of view transducers have a more complicated geometry and electronics and are likely to, in the future, bridge the gap between hand-held transducers and whole breast scanners. Such spatial orientation can be invaluable to the treating clinician.

RECENT TECHNICAL DEVELOPMENTS

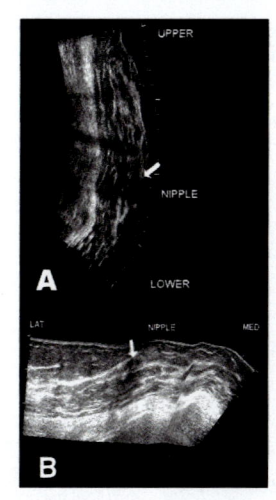

Fig. 3.6: Long transducers with a large number of transducer elements can function as combined linear arrays in the central portion and phased array in the peripheral part to yield a virtual large field of view. These transducers are hand held and are moved mechanically over the zone of interest. Information can be obtained in a large number of planes (A and B)

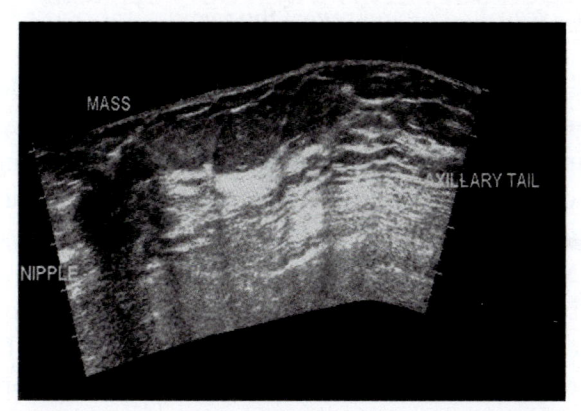

Fig. 3.7: Extended field of view studies are very useful for displaying the localization of a mass within the breast and are greatly appreciated by the treating surgeon

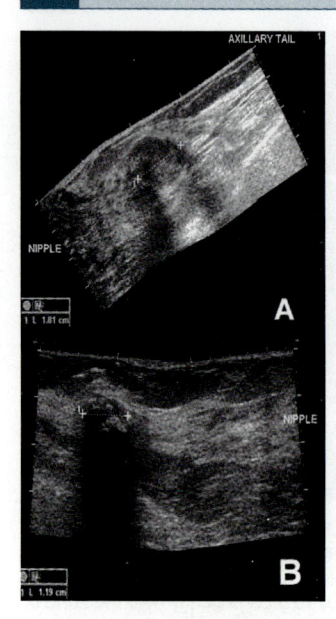

Fig. 3.8: The ability to display spatial relationships within the breast improves conceptualisation of normal and abnormal tissues and helps in planning and executing optimal surgical technique. Extended field of view studies as shown in these two patients (A and B) are an ideal display format for this purpose

COLOUR DOPPLER, POWER DOPPLER AND SPECTRAL DOPPLER

The use of flow studies, both morphology and flow characteristics, remains an integral part of the breast examination. Although no clear indices and guidelines are currently apparent, certain indicators are becoming apparent in recent literature:
- Many breast cancers are poorly vascular as are benign lesions; this is because vascularity is not a consequence of malignancy per se but a result of rate of tumour growth, cellularity and host response
- Negative end-diastolic velocities are often seen in malignant lesions (Figs 3.9 and 3.10). Unlike other

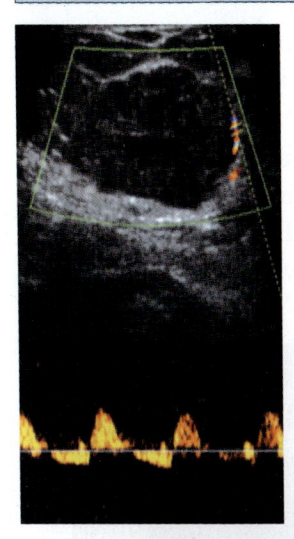

Fig. 3.9: Unlike other organs where malignant tumoral neoangiogenesis is characterised by a low impedance flow and vessels where the media is muscle deprived, in the breast malignant tumours often display negative end-diastolic velocities

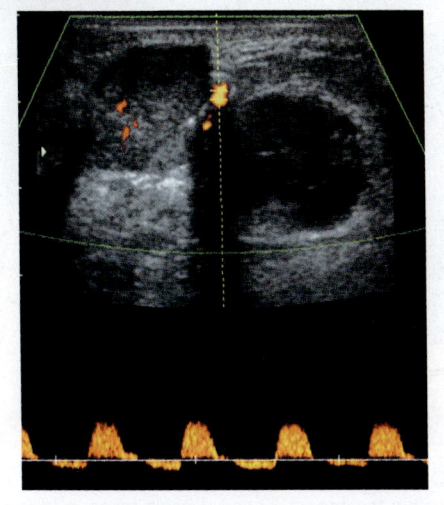

Fig. 3.10: In lesions which have unconvincing malignant characteristics of the margins, shape and echogenecity, colour Doppler spectra with negative end-diastolic velocities are useful pointers for a possible malignant process

organs where muscle-poor neoangiogenesis vessels are low impedance high diastolic flow circuits, in the breast this is often a marker of benign disease and is a consequence of an inflammatory response to degeneration (Figs 3.11 and 3.12)
- Sensitivity is markedly different on high end equipment compared to low end equipment

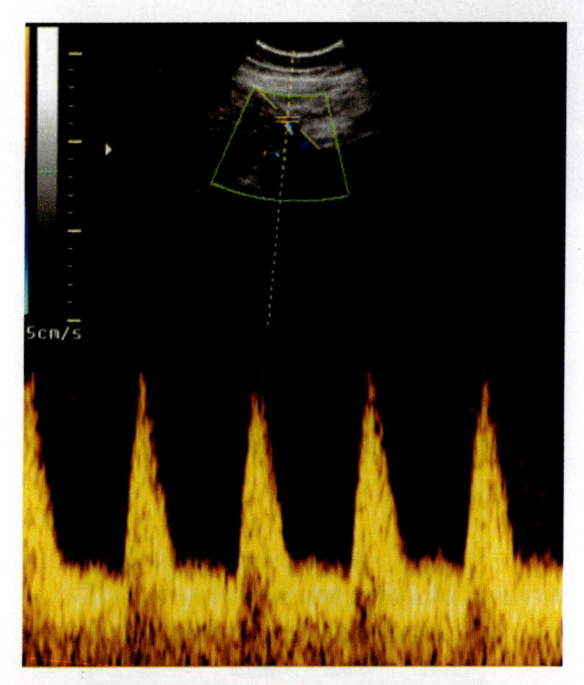

Fig. 3.11: Degeneration in benign masses often excites an inflammatory response within the breast. These vessels reveal a high diastolic flow low impedance flow velocity waveform akin to malignant vessels in other organs

RECENT TECHNICAL DEVELOPMENTS 31

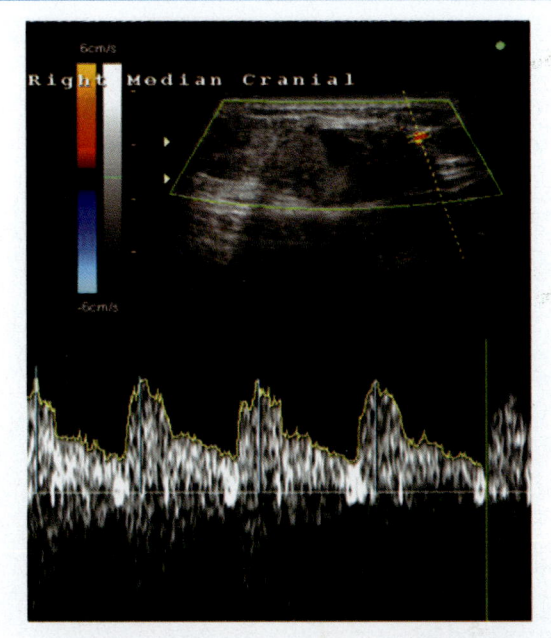

Fig. 3.12: Heteroechoic fibroadenoma showing a low impedance flow velocity waveform

- Beam steering markedly reduces sensitivity
- Colour flow can help differentiate the cause of internal echoes in a focal lesion; debris of any origin is avascular and vessels indicate live tissue (Fig. 3.13)
- Power Doppler is angle independent and shows very slow flow making it ideal for assessing neo-angiogenesis.

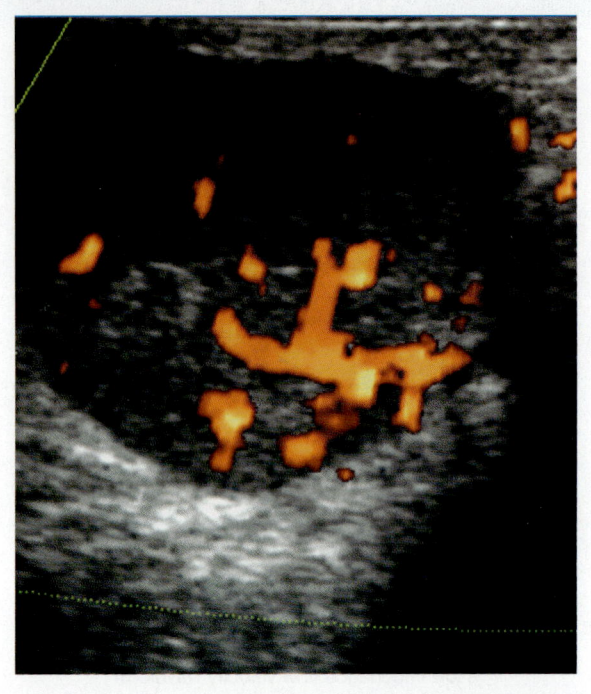

Fig. 3.13: Echogenic material within lesion can represent cellular debris or tissues. The presence of vascular signals in the contents of a lesion indicates that the lesion contains live tissue. This "echogenic cyst" revealed vascular signals. Sampling showed an invasive lobular carcinoma

Chapter 4

Anatomical Considerations

STEP BY STEP BREAST ULTRASOUND

The breast is only roughly globular in shape.
- The *nipple* lies slightly medial and inferior to the geometric centre of the breast (Fig. 4.1). The upper outer quadrant of each breast, therefore, has more breast tissue and this is one of the reasons for more breast lesions in this area. The other reason is the slower regression of tissues in this area with age.
- Breast tissue extends into the axilla (Fig. 4.2). This is called the *tail* of the breast. This is also called the axillary segment or tail of Spence.

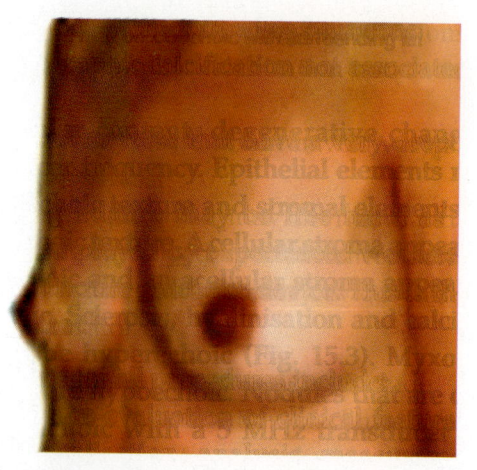

Fig. 4.1: The nipple is not located in the centre of the breast. It is usually located medial and inferior to the geometric centre of the breast

ANATOMICAL CONSIDERATIONS 35

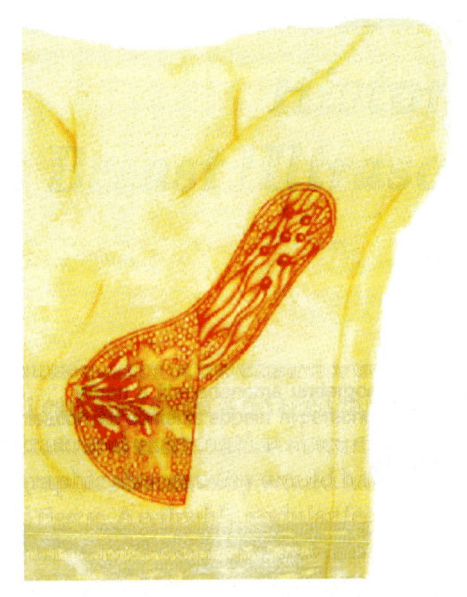

Fig. 4.2: The breast tissue extends into the axilla. This is also known as the axillary segment or tail of the breast

- *Accessory breast* tissue (Fig. 4.3) is not unusual in occurrence and is usually found in the axilla. It may also occur in the upper outer quadrants or in the 6:00 position adjacent to breast tissue and cause asymmetry or a palpable lump. It may also occur anywhere along the milk line.
- Each breast consists of 15-20 *lobes* (Fig. 4.4). Each lobe consists of *lobules* and *branch ducts* (Fig. 4.5). Branch ducts join to form *larger ducts*. These converge to form one *main subareolar duct* which drains the whole lobe. Each lobar duct widens just deep to the nipple.

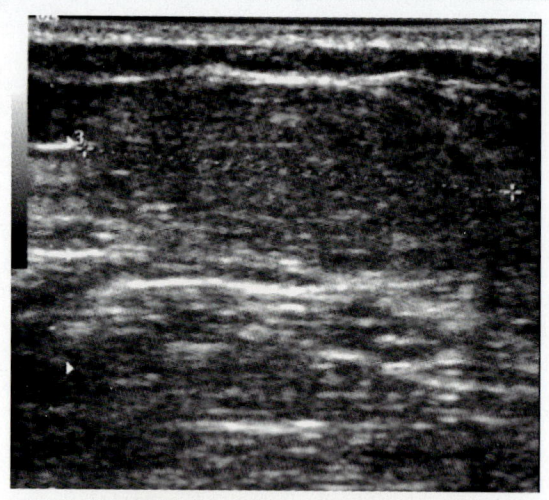

Fig. 4.3: Accessory breast tissue is usually found in the axilla. It almost always consists of ovoid glandular element echoes with a thin-echogenic capsule

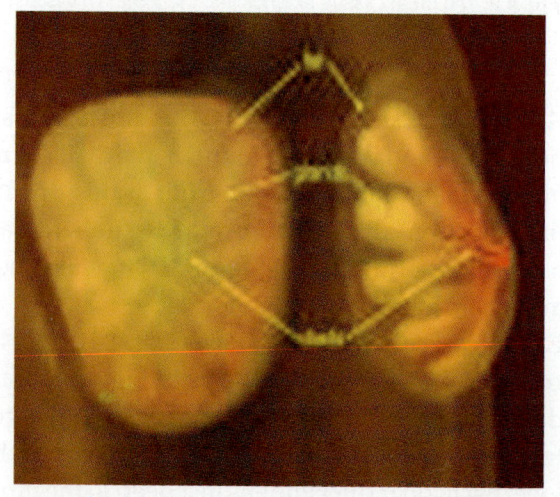

Fig. 4.4: Each breast consists of 15-20 lobes

ANATOMICAL CONSIDERATIONS 37

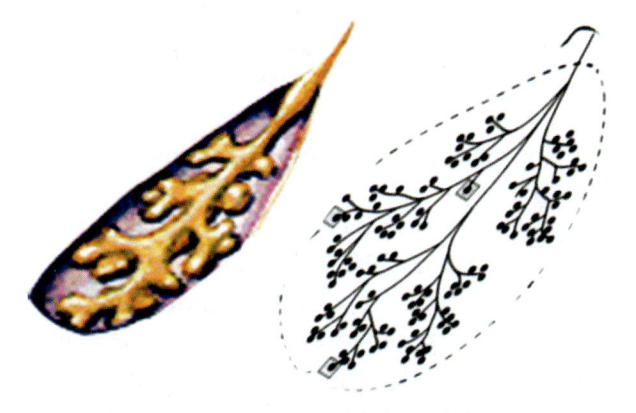

Fig. 4.5: Each lobe consists of lobules and branch ducts. Branch ducts join to form larger ducts. These have a radial orientation

This is known as a *lactiferous sinus*. Some main subareolar ducts converge before reaching the nipple. There are, therefore, fewer duct orifices than lobes.

- Larger ducts have a *radial orientation*. Tortuosity may give them other orientations. Smaller branch ducts have a non-radial orientation but very small ones may be oriented radially again. Lobar ducts tend to lie nearer to the chest wall than to the skin. This is because more lobules arise anteriorly and anterolaterally than on their posterior aspect. The orientation of anterior and anterolateral lobules accounts for the vertical orientation of most small breast cancers.

Breast tissue lies between the *skin* and the *chest wall*. There are three sonographically distinct zones in the breast (Fig. 4.6). From superficial to deep, these are:
- The premammary or *subcutaneous zone*, consisting of fat, suspensory (Cooper's) ligaments and blood vessels.
- The *mammary zone* which is encompassed by the premammary fascia anteriorly and the retromammary fascia posteriorly. Almost all of the mammary ducts and lobules lie in this zone, which also contains stromal fat, fibrous tissue and extensions of suspensory ligaments.

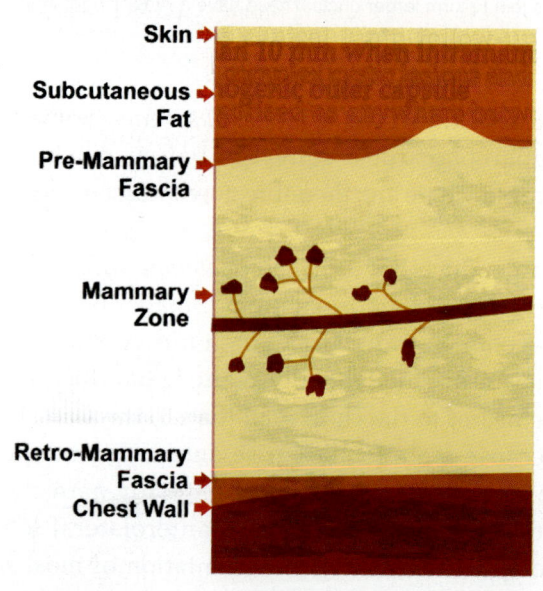

Fig. 4.6: Schematic representation of breast tissue

ANATOMICAL CONSIDERATIONS

- The *retromammary zone* contains mainly fat and some suspensory ligaments. This zone lies anterior to the pectoralis major muscle.

Breasts may show a predominantly glandular, predominantly fatty or a mixed echo pattern (Figs 4.7 to 4.9).

Terminal ductolobular units (TDLUs) are the functional units of the breast (Fig. 4.10).
- Each consists of a lobule and its terminal duct.
- Hundreds and even thousands of these are present in each breast.

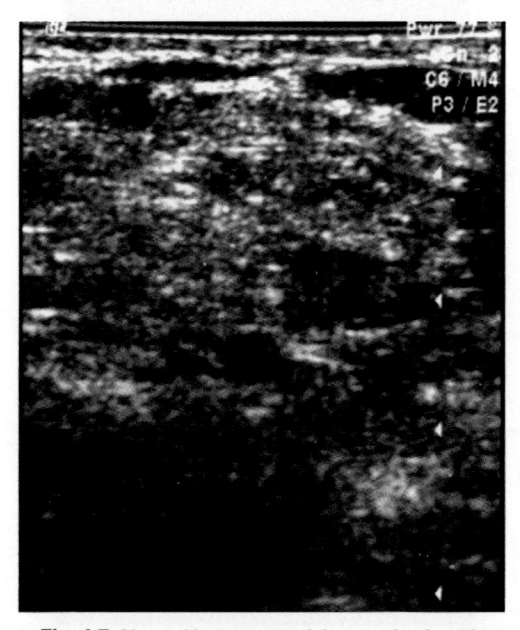

Fig. 4.7: Normal breast containing predominantly glandular elements

40 STEP BY STEP BREAST ULTRASOUND

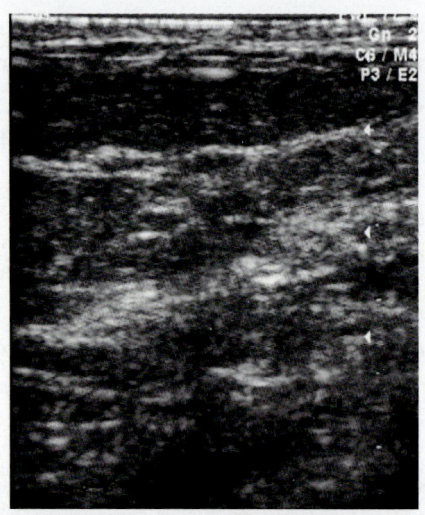

Fig. 4.8: Normal breast showing predominantly fatty elements

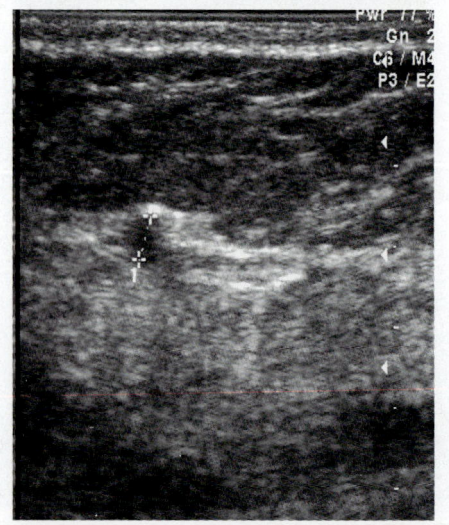

Fig. 4.9: Breast showing an equivalent of fatty and glandular elements and a small haemorrhagic cyst

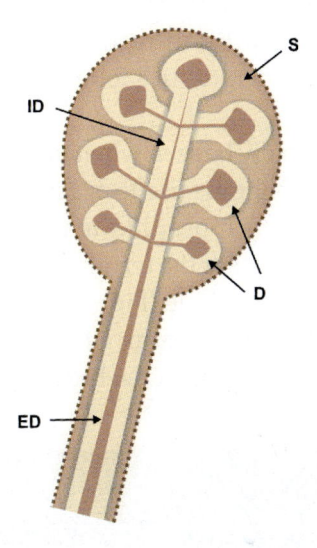

Fig. 4.10: Terminal ductolobular unit. ED: Extralobular terminal duct, ID: Intralobular terminal duct, D: Ductules, S: Intralobular fibrous stroma

- This is the site of origin of most breast pathology.
- TDLUs usually arise from peripheral branch ducts but may arise from larger central ducts.
- Proliferate rapidly during adolescence and in the early third decade, in pregnancy and lactation, in the post-ovulatory phase of each cycle, with hormone replacement therapy (HRT) and with exogenous oestrogen as in contraceptive pills.
- Regression is rapid after pregnancy and in menopause and often asymmetric, both within the breast and between right and left.

- Cannot be seen by ultrasound in most patients because all structures in a lobule are isoechoic with each other.
- May occasionally be seen when they are surrounded by echogenic fibrous tissue or fat.
- When seen, they appear like tennis rackets with the handle representing the terminal duct and the head representing the lobule (Fig. 4.11).
- Size varies from 1-7 mm. Enlarged TDLUs may obscure small lesions in the breast.

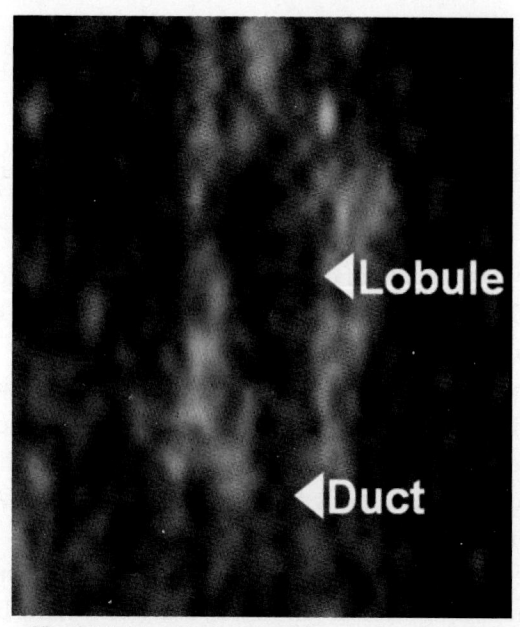

Fig. 4.11: Magnified ultrasound image of a normal terminal ductolobular unit (TDLU)

ANATOMICAL CONSIDERATIONS 43

LYMPHATIC DRAINAGE

The breast drains largely into a rich layer of lymphatics just superficial to the anterior mammary fascia (Fig. 4.12). From here the drainage proceeds to the periareolar plexus and then mainly to the axilla. Minimal drainage takes place to the internal mammary and infraclavicular lymph nodes.

The presence of diseased nodes, their number and level is a key prognostic indicator in breast cancer. An attempt to delineate this should, therefore, be made when the breast is evaluated.

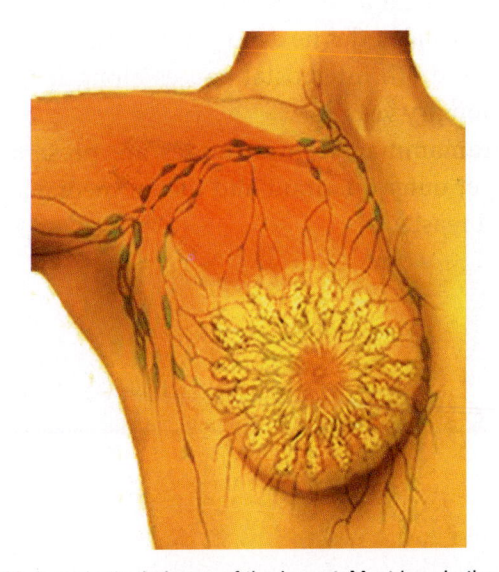

Fig. 4.12: Lymphatic drainage of the breast. Most lymphatics of the breast first drain to just superficial to the anterior mammary fascia and then to the periareolar plexus and the axilla. Some lymphatics drain into the internal mammary and infraclavicular lymph nodes

Axillary lymph nodes are categorised on the basis of their location with respect to the pectoralis minor muscle.
- Level I nodes lie lateral and inferior to the pectoralis minor
- Level II lie deep to the pectoralis minor
- Level III lie medial and superior to the pectoralis minor muscle
- Sentinel node evaluation involves the lowest of level I nodes
- Axillary dissections involve level I and level II nodes
- Radical mastectomy and modified radical mastectomies include removals of levels I and II
- Intercostal nodes lie deep to the sternum in the 2nd, 3rd and 4th intercostal spaces along the internal mammary vessels
- Intramammary lymph nodes are present in the upper outer quadrant and the far medial aspect of the breast.

Chapter 5
Patient Positioning

Unlike mammography, breast ultrasound can be optimised by changing patient position and adjusting patient position to improve visualisation in various parts of the breast.

- With the patient *supine*, the ipsilateral arm is abducted and the elbow flexed to bring the *hand below the head* (Fig. 5.1). This thins and flattens the breast. This is the usual position for assessing the inner quadrants.
- To assess the outer quadrants it is often necessary to use a *contralateral posterior oblique* posture (Fig. 5.2). In this, the breast to be scanned is elevated relative to the opposite breast. The usual elevation is 30-45

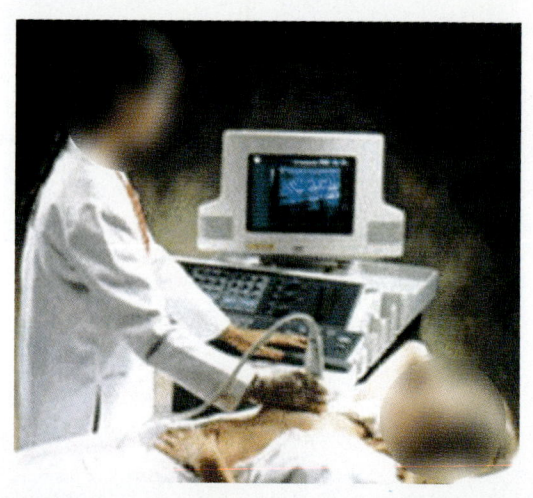

Fig. 5.1: Most breasts can be evaluated in the supine position as shown. This makes the breast flat and thin and allows the beam of high frequency transducer to penetrate upto the chest wall. Additional positions are required for larger breasts

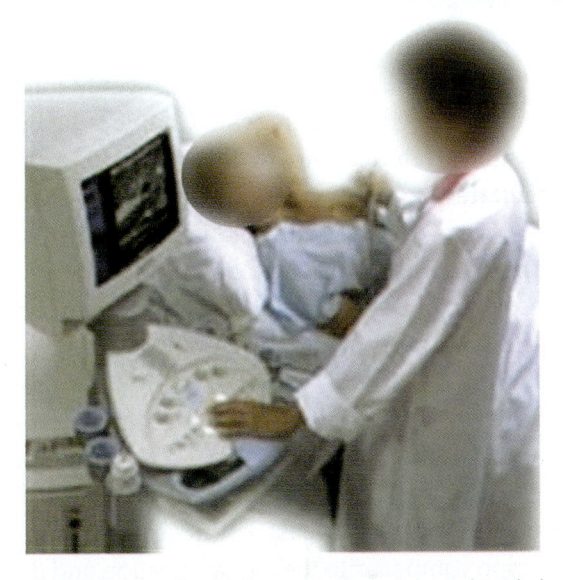

Fig. 5.2: In order to adequately assess the outer quadrant in larger breasts it is useful to employ a contralateral posterior oblique position. The breast to be examined is elevated relative to the opposite breast by 30-45 degrees. The larger the breast and the closer the lesion to the axilla, the greater the obliquity require for better penetration of a high frequency near field focused ultrasound beam

degrees. Obliquity needs to be varied depending on breast size, pendulousness and location of lesion. The larger and more pendulous the breast the greater the obliquity required. The more lateral the region of interest, the greater the degree of obliquity required. This position thins out the breast and permits better penetration of the breast by a high frequency near field focussed beam. Stretching of the breast in this position tends to *stretch out wrinkles* in the skin of the breast and this prevents trapping of air bubbles during the scan. Cooper's ligaments also get stretched out in this position and this facilitates the ability to compress a lesion between the skin and chest wall. Obliquity also puts the normally conically oriented tissues of the breast into a horizontal orientation. This minimises critical angle shadowing and prevents degradation of focussing.

- If a lesion is palpable in an *upright* position only, examination should be carried out in an upright position as well. This is particularly useful for superficial lesions. The breast is thicker in an upright position compared to the supine position and deeper lesions may be missed completely if the examination is performed in an upright position only.
- *Central ducts* are often seen well in an upright position because their tortuosity is often straightened out in this position.
- *Movement of debris* can be demonstrated by scanning in changing positions. This is useful not only in haemorrhagic or inflammatory lesions but in assessing milk of magnesium and fat-fluid levels as well.
- The *sub-areolar nipple complex* requires special attention. Cold room and cold jelly temperatures cause myoepithelial elements in the breast to contract, thereby wrinkling the area and causing critical angle shadowing. This can be avoided by

scanning in a warm room and by using a large blob of warm jelly. Placing the transducer at the edge of the nipple and angling to the retroareolar region may better demonstrate this area.

It is worth noting that unlike mammography, ultrasound identifies the location of a lesion in the same postures as those employed by a surgeon, thereby, enhancing clinical and imaging correlation.

Chapter 6
Scanning Techniques

Technique is as important to breast ultrasound as technically superior equipment.

TRANSDUCER CONSIDERATIONS

7.5-12 MHz transducers penetrate most breasts. A lower frequency may be used in:
- Very large breasts
- Very obese women
- Very large implants
- Severe lymphoedema or inflammation of the breast.

Acoustic power should be turned up to a maximum before changing to a lower frequency transducer.

Most manufacturers now offer electronic focussing of beams along the long axis during both transmit and receive phases. This greatly improves lateral resolution.

SCANNING PLANES

Real time scans may be performed longitudinally or transversely or both. The process should be akin to lawn-mowing with each strip minimally overlapping the previous one. The survey can also be done in a radial direction, an antiradial direction or both. Ductal anatomy requires scanning in radial planes.

SIMULTANEOUS PALPATION AND SCANNING

This is an invaluable tool to assess palpable abnormalities and greatly increases the yield of a diagnosis. It ensures that a palpable lesion is neither missed nor over diagnosed.

MAMMOGRAPHIC CORRELATION

Location of a lesion does not coincide exactly with conventional mammography. 6:00 and 12:00 locations coincide largely. Other locations will vary depending on the angle of the X-Ray beam. It is wise to have mammography films available for a review when an ultrasound is carried out and vice versa.

SPLIT SCREEN IMAGE

These are useful for:
- Mirror-image correlations
- Documenting dynamic events without the cumbersome video record method
- Assessing compressibility
- Assessing mobility
- Demonstration of movement in lesions that contain debris
- Evaluating subareolar ducts.

SCAN SPEEDS

Rapid scanning can obscure small lesions. It is important to go slow as this gives an enhanced yield of diagnosis. One way to avoid rapid scanning is to use four focal zones. With this, the frame rate goes down, resolution improves and the image gets blurred if the transducer is moved too fast.

COMPRESSION

All breast lesions should be re-evaluated with compression. Compression thins breast tissue, improves penetration and enhances image quality. This is particularly useful for lesions near the chest wall. Sometimes, compression works the opposite way by producing near field reverberations and side lobe artefacts deep inside breast tissue.

FREMITUS

When the patient hums or says eeeeee, the tissues in and around a lesion will vibrate depending on their elasticity. This is called fremitus and can be observed as a power Doppler map during ultrasound. This can be used for differentiating normal fat from a true nodule, the amount of spiculation surrounding a solid mass, to identify multifocal disease and to increase the index of suspicion in solid masses.

Chapter 7

Annotating Lesion Location

Documenting the location of a lesion is important because:
- It permits locating the lesion for ultrasound-guided punctures at a later date
- It allows more accurate comparison in follow-up studies
- It is an easy-to-use method to use during the scan and uses fewer key-strokes.

We use a five component code to describe location:
- The first notation is the side, left or right, abbreviated L or R
- The second is a clock-face position. Half-way positions may be used when necessary.
- The third notation is a scan-plane orientation (Fig. 7.1): longitudinal (LO), transverse (TR), radial (RAD), antiradial (AR) or oblique (OBL).
- The fourth notation is depth of the lesion (Fig. 7.2). This may be expressed in centimetres or as A, B or C, where each zone represents one-third of the breast thickness. A is most superficial, B is the middle zone and C is the zone near the chest wall. Most pathological lesions arise in zone B.
- The fifth notation is distance from the nipple (Fig. 7.3). This is done by mentioning the distance in centimetres or by notations 1, 2, 3, SA (subareolar) or A (axillary). The breast is divided into three equally wide concentric rings from the nipple to the periphery. The inner ring is 1, the middle one 2 and the outer one 3. Because of the changes in position

ANNOTATING LESION LOCATION

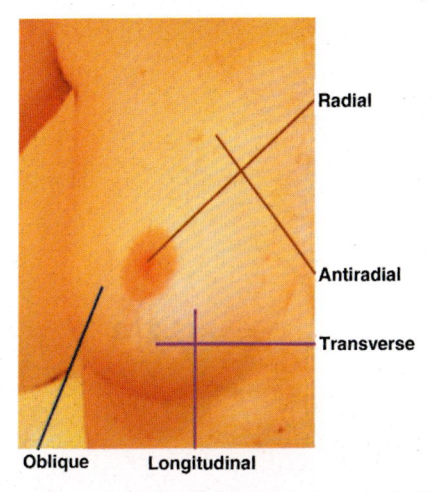

Fig. 7.1: Scan plane orientation. This forms an important of the notation of a lesion and is expressed as the orientation of the long axis of a lesion within the breast: longitudinal (LO), transverse (TR), Radial (RAD), antiradial (AR) and oblique (OBL)

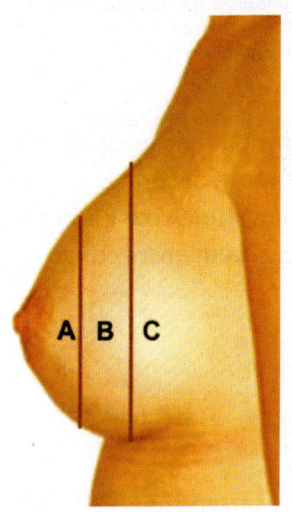

Fig. 7.2: The depth of a lesion within the breast may be expressed in centimetres or as A, B or C where each zone represents one-third of the thickness of entire breast. A is most superficial, B is the middle zone and C is the area just anterior to the chest wall

58 STEP BY STEP BREAST ULTRASOUND

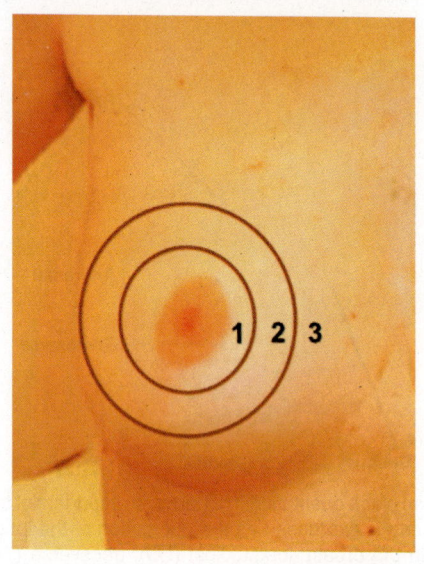

Fig. 7.3: Distance of a lesion from a nipple is either expressed in centimetres or as 1, 2 or 3. The breast is divided into three concentric rings from the nipple to the periphery. 1 is the inner ring, 2 is the middle ring and 3 is the outer ring

with breast compression and patient position, the actual distance notation is more accurate. It is of course more cumbersome and time-consuming to use, because the actual measurement needs to be taken with a scale.

Chapter 8
Echogenecity

Although breast lesions have been labelled as *hypoechoic*, *hyperechoic* and *isoechoic* since the inception of gray scale ultrasound, older literature did not set any standard breast or chest wall tissue or organ against which these echo-intensities were or could be compared.

In relatively more recent years, normal *interlobular dense stromal fibrous tissue* has been considered the standard for comparison. Unfortunately, this lies almost at one end of the echogenic spectrum and only *microcalcifications* and *needles* are more echogenic. Additionally, all other pathologic lesions and all other normal breast tissue would be hypoechoic and, therefore, the ability to differentiate and reassess descriptions is not objective enough.

It was then realised that it would be logical and practical to choose a *standard of reference* which is:
- Represented by a normal, universally found component of breast tissue
- Located at the centre of the gray scale.

The choice was therefore, limited to one of three:
- Fatty elements
- TDLUs
- Ductal and periductal tissues.

Since *TDLUs* and *ductal and periductal tissue* are not always demonstrable in all patients and *fat* is seen in virtually all breasts, it is being increasingly accepted as a standard for comparing normal and abnormal echogenecities in the breast (Fig. 8.1). Most workers

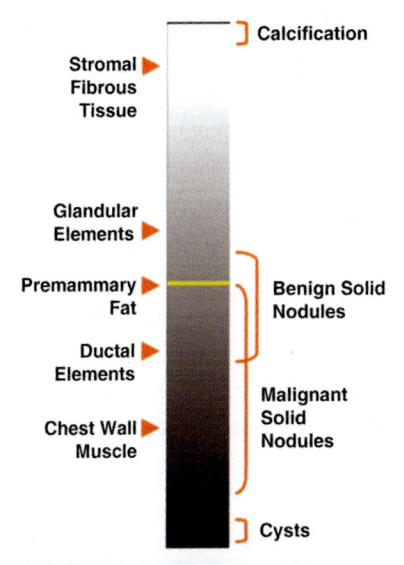

Fig. 8.1: Since all breasts have fatty elements, the echogenecity of fat is now being increasingly used as a reference standard for a semi-quantification of the echogenecity of normal and abnormal breast components. Most lesions are less than echogenic than fat. Intensely echogenic interlobular fibrous stroma has for many years been used as a reference. Using this, however, reduces the range of grays against which all other tissues can be compared and therefore the shift to fat as a midpoint reference

have now changed to comparing normal and pathologic structures with subcutaneous or premammary zone fat and the settings on the equipment, therefore, are appropriately changed to make fat appear as a midlevel gray and not black or hypoechoic. Since most lesions are hypoechoic with reference to fat, their distinctness will be reduced if fat is made hypoechoic to midlevel grays. To achieve this midlevel gray appearance of fat it is necessary to adjust the *total gain* and the *time-gain curve (TGC)* as well. It is equally important to ensure that fat throughout the breast, whether subcutaneous, premammary or retromammary should have the same midlevel gray echogenecity (Fig. 8.2). The TGC that is appropriate is usually mildly sloping. A *flat TGC* makes subcutaneous fat hyperechoic and retromammary fat too hypoechoic. A *steep TGC* will have the opposite effect.

An overview of echogenecity of normal breast tissues, benign breast conditions and neoplastic lesions is given below.

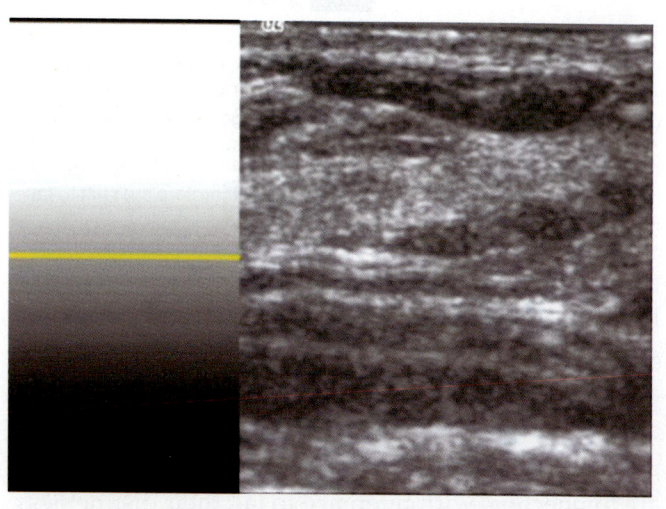

Fig. 8.2: Ideal gray scale settings for breast ultrasound

Isoechoic Tissues

- Fat
- Ductules in TDLUs
- Intralobular fibrous stroma
- Periductal fibrous stroma
- Papillary apocrine metaplasia
- Debris in cysts
- Adenosis
- Floral/papillary/duct hyperplasia
- Papillomas
- Adenomas
- Some carcinomas.

Anechoic Tissues

- Clear cyst contents
- Fluid in ducts
- Most lymphatics
- Cystic necrosis in tumours
- Most lymphomas
- Medullary carcinomas.

Hypoechoic Tissues

- Nipple
- Haematomas
- Abscesses
- Debris in ducts
- Most carcinomas
- Medullary carcinoma.

Hyperechoic Tissues

- Skin
- Cooper's ligaments
- Interlobular fibrous stroma
- Cyst walls
- Pseudocapsules
- Fibrosis
- Oedema of fat
- Central scars in carcinomas
- Haloes in carcinomas
- Post-needling.

A critical appraisal of this list brings to the fore several aspects of ultrasound delineation and characterisation of tissues. A largely hyperechoic fibrous breast will offer the highest sensitivity for lesions, close to 100%. A largely isoechoic glandular breast tissue will offer the least sensitivity, but this is still satisfactory as it is about 90%. Fortunately, most breasts have a mixture of hyperechoic fibrous tissue and isoechoic glandular tissue which offers a reasonable sensitivity to identify pathology. Importantly, ultrasound can distinctly differentiate the mammographically dense breast into three types: purely isoechoic glandular tissue, purely hyperechoic fibrous tissue, and a mixture of both these types.

Chapter 9

Reporting and Communication

Basic ultrasound characterisation of clinically palpable or mammographically delineated breast masses divides lesions into any of the following categories:
- Normal tissue
- Simple cystic lesion
- Complex cystic lesion
- Solid lesions.

A second, more relevant, level of characterisation places each lesion into a risk category for malignancy. This second level categorisation has been suggested by Stavros and co-workers from the United States of America and is becoming widely known as the Ultrasound BIRADS categorisation. BIRADS stands for Breast Imaging Reporting and Data System. The categories are based on the BIRADS mammographic risk categories suggested by the American College of Radiology. Table 9.1 shows the ACR BIRADS categorisation and Table 9.2 shows the Ultrasound BIRADS recommendations.

The aim of the Ultrasound BIRADS categorisation is the same as the Mammographic BIRADS categorisation and includes the following:
- To standardise terminology
- To make sonologists commit themselves in the official report
- To prevent unclear reports
- To reduce intra-operator variability
- To create user-friendly databases
- Improve internal and outsider audits.

REPORTING AND COMMUNICATION

Table 9.1: Americal college of radiology breast imaging reporting and data system (BIRADS) mammographic risk categories

BIRADS category	Description	Risk of malignancy (%)	Management
0	Incomplete, needs additional evaluation	Uncertain	Diagnostic mammograms, ultrasound etc.
1	Normal	0	Return to routine screening
2	Benign finding	0	Return to routine screening
3	Probably benign	≤ 2	Patient choice: follow-up versus biopsy
4	Suspicious	> 2 and < 90	Biopsy
5	Malignant	≥ 90	Biopsy

Table 9.2: Modified american college of radiology breast imaging reporting and data system (BIRADS) ultrasound risk categories

BIRADS category	Description	Risk of malignancy (%)	Management
1	Normal	0	Clinical lump follow up and return to screening
2	Benign finding	0	Clinical lump follow up and return to screening
3	Probably benign	≤ 2	Patient choice: follow up versus biopsy
4a	Mildly suspicious	> 2 and < 50	Biopsy (additional imaging?)
4b	Moderately suspicious	> 50 and < 90	Biopsy
5	Malignant	≥ 90	Biopsy

Although both the mammographic and the Ultrasound BIRADS categorisations are not yet foolproof in their application, they represent a major step forward towards an objective management of breast lesions. Importantly, they reduce subjective bias in assessing breast lesions and, at the same time, keep a reasonable perspective of the perils and unpleasantries of litigation.

When a palpable lesion shows normal sonoanatomy the lesion is labelled as Ultrasound BIRADS 1 and needs a clinical follow-up and screening as per conventional mammographic criteria, i.e. patient age, family history, previous lesions, etc.

Simple cysts are categorised as Ultrasound BIRADS 2 which again implies clinical lump follow-up and return to screening. All complex cystic lesions and solid lesions should be categorised as anywhere between 2 and 5 to facilitate management decisions. This implies a patient option between biopsy and clinical follow-up for Ultrasound BIRADS 3 lesions and biopsy of all Ultrasound BIRADS 4 and 5 lesions. Category 4 has been subdivided into a and b for medicolegal considerations since the word "probable" has an implied incidence of 50% or more in legal parlance. Category 4a implies a risk of more than 2% and less than 50% and category 4b implies a risk of more than 50% and less than 90%. All lesions that are considered at a risk of 90 to 100% for malignancy are categorised as Ultrasound BIRADS 5.

REPORTING AND COMMUNICATION

Each lesion in each breast should have an Ultrasound BIRADS categorisation. The overall Ultrasound BIRADS category is the highest category of any of the lesions in that breast. For instance, if a breast has three palpable abnormalities and these correspond to one area of normal glandular tissue (Ultrasound BIRADS 1), one simple cyst (Ultrasound BIRADS 2) and a shaggy vascular cyst (Ultrasound BIRADS 5) the overall category is Ultrasound BIRADS 5.

As a consequence of the existence of the Ultrasound BIRADS 1 category there is no such thing as a negative breast ultrasound examination since every palpable or mammographic abnormality would have an equivalent of normal tissue. A palpable nodular feel corresponding to normal glandular tissue, for example would reassure the patient and the clinician of the lesion being a variant of norm and not a doubtful abnormality being missed on the examination and therefore requiring a biopsy.

Preliminary studies reveal that as a consequence of Ultrasound BIRADS categorisation:
- Biopsy rates are reduced for categories 1-4
- Pick-up rates of category 5 lesions is enhanced compared to mammography
- A larger number of lesions are appropriately down-categorised to 1.

Extensive use of Ultrasound has also shown that mammograms are frequently negative in patients with palpable lumps consequent to non-neoplastic fibroglandular ridges. An Ultrasound BIRADS categorisation conveniently and correctly puts these fibroglandular ridges in Category 1. Equally importantly, ultrasound better delineates multifocal disease, extraductal spread of lesions, and, lymph node disease.

Chapter 10

Interventional Procedures

The rapidly expanding list of ultrasound guided needle procedures includes the following:
- Cyst aspiration
- Aspiration biopsies
- Abscess drainage
- Mammotomy
- Needle localisation
- Ductography
- Radiofrequency and laser tumour ablations
- Sentinel node analysis.

Ultrasound is the modality of choice for all guided procedures except the following situations:
- Mammographic calcification not associated with a mass
- Very small nodules that have a very deep location in large breasts.

Needle guidance may be free hand as is more frequently employed by experienced workers or may be with a puncture guidance device. This is the choice of the operator.

General steps for all procedures include:
- Thorough re-evaluation of clinical features, ultrasound localisation, analysis, measurement and documentation
- Review of mammograms when available
- Informed consent including simple aspects of haemorrhage, pain, sepsis, failure to obtain an adequate sample, failure to supply an accurate report and anaesthetic complications

INTERVENTIONAL PROCEDURES

- Positioning the patient as for breast ultrasound
- Reevaluation of the lesion just prior to puncture
- Transducer sterilisation using a sterile cover or chemical cleaning
- Sterile ultrasound gel
- Confirming that needles fit the puncture guidance device if one is being used
- Skin preparation
- Continuous communication with the patient
- Confirming the adequacy of the sample with the pathologist.

Two general approaches are used: short axis or long axis. The former uses a shortest distance method by passing the needle adjacent to the transducer with least extent of passage through breast tissue. The angle of the needle may be steep or shallow. The skin puncture may be juxta-transducer or at a short distance. The advantage lies in quick access but suffers from a lack of continuous needle length visualization. In a long axis approach the needle is passed perpendicular to the transducer axis and can be seen along its entire length.

The mammosound is an automated prone digital ultrasound stereotactic biopsy table with integrated and correlated automated ultrasound.

Three dimensional (3D) and real time Three dimensional (4D) ultrasound is greatly expanding the sensitivity of the technique to an accurate diagnosis and better interventional guidance.

CYST ASPIRATION

Aspiration of a breast cyst is not necessary for diagnosis. It is useful in the following situations:
- Relief of pain
- Relief of anxiety
- To compare with previous puncture yield
- Recurrent cysts.

Needles frequently used include a 21 gauge vacutainer system or a 16 gauge needle if the lesion is at depth.

ABSCESS DRAINAGE

This has emerged as the single most important method of treating a breast cyst. Aspirates should always be sent for cytology and microbial evaluation. Short-term catheter drainage is not a current practice. Intralesional antibiotic injections are not usually required.

DUCTOGRAPHY

This involves assessing the duct that cannot be cannulated and a detailed breast evaluation.

BIOPSIES

Three kinds of biopsies exist: Fine Needle Aspiration Biopsy, Automated Large Core Biopsy, and Directional Vacuum assisted Biopsy (Mammotomy).

16 or 18 gauge ultrasound guided biopsies of the breast have been around for many years but suffer from

the disadvantage of being cytology and not histology based. They are gradually falling out of flavor.

Automated Large Core Devices are commercially available. The advantage lies in obtaining tissue cores which yield a better diagnosis. 5-6 cores can be obtained and assessed. Coaxial needles are available as well.

Directional Vacuum Assisted Biopsy or mammotomy is a cutting technique guided by ultrasound. The device is handheld and guided to just posterior to the lesion and then a scooping out is carried out.

RADIOFREQUENCY ABLATION

Pulsed radiofrequency devices can be used to ablate tumours. Results from recent trials are encouraging and federal approval is awaited.

Section 3

Benign and Malignant Lesions

Chapter 11

Development and Involution

The vast majority of women presenting with breast symptoms have benign breast disease, particularly in the developed world. These patients usually have breast pain, breast cysts or fibroadenomas.

Over the past years there has been a quantum leap in the understanding of normal and aberrant breast development and this has improved the interpretation of mammograms and breast ultrasound.

Many disorders are no longer regarded as disease entities and have been reclassified as "aberrations of normal development and involution (ANDI)". Disorders of development include fibroadenomas and juvenile hypertrophy. Disorders of involution include cysts, duct ectasia and mild epithelial hyperplasia. Cyclical and secretory changes include nodularity and cyclical mastalgia.

Up to the age of 25 years there is an early reproductive phase of breast development characterized by stromal development and the formation of ducts and lobules. Fibroadenomas are most common during this period. This phase is also commonly marked by the variable appearance and disappearance of breast nodularity associated with breast pain, duct papillomas causing a nipple discharge and galactoceles during lactation. The 25-40-year-old age group goes through a mature reproductive phase of breast development. An

DEVELOPMENT AND INVOLUTION

involutional or degenerative phase is seen in women beyond the age of 40. Breast cysts, sclerosing lesions, duct ectasia and hyperplasia occur more frequently during this degenerative phase. Increased use of hormone replacement therapy in the involutional phase has led to an increase in the incidence of breast pain in this age group.

The ANDI classification helps in understanding the spectrum of disorders. The relative risk of breast cancer is, however, evident from the Dupont and Page classification which classifies these lesions as simple cysts with no increased risk, proliferative change without atypia such as sclerosing adenosis which has only a minimally increased risk, and proliferative changes with atypia such as atypical ductal hyperplasia (ADH), which have a four- to five-fold increase in the relative risk of breast cancer.

Fibrocystic change (FCC) arises most frequently in the TDLUs and rarely from centrally located ducts. It has two components, variable from patient to patient, from one breast to another, from one lobule to the next and within a lobule as well. The two components include dilatation and effacement of the ductal elements (Fig. 11.1) and hyalinization and sclerosis of intralobular stromal tissue. The former presents as cysts and the latter as hyperechoic enlargement of the TDLU

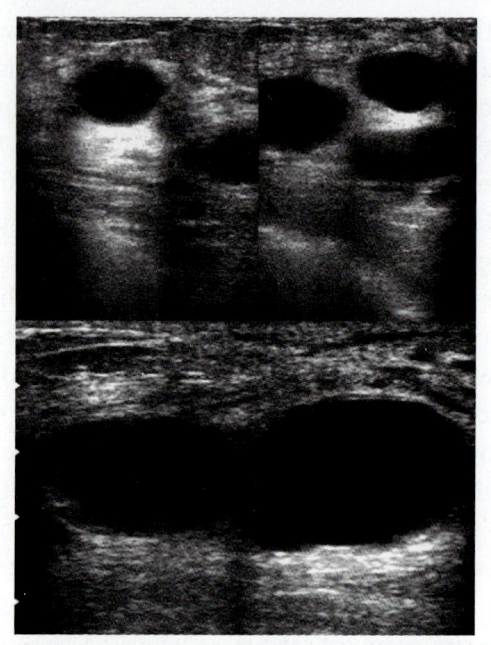

Fig. 11.1: Fibrocystic change usually arises in the TDLU. Dilatation and effacement of ductal element results in the formation of thin-walled cysts

(Fig. 11.2). Changes are easier to characterise when affected TDLUs are imaged along their long axis.

When dilated TDLUs become distended with material they can present as solid (Fig. 11.3) and not cystic lesions. The material that can cause this solid appearance can include the following: papillary apocrine metaplasia, duct hyperplasia, sclerosing adenosis, fibrosis, foamy macrophages, and blood cells. Cysts less than 1-2 mm can sometimes not be resolved and may present as echogenic nodules.

DEVELOPMENT AND INVOLUTION 83

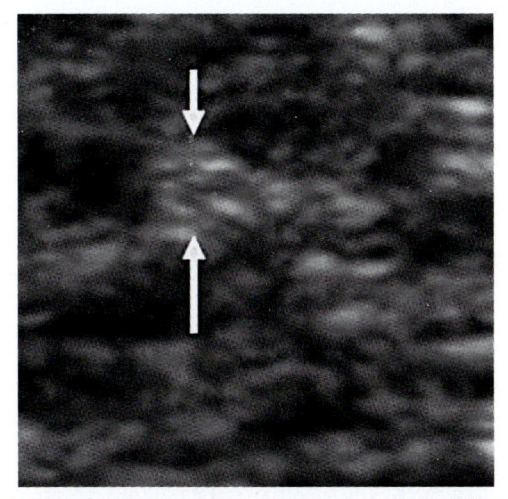

Fig. 11.2: When the predominant pathologic process in fibrocystic change is hyalinization and sclerosis of intralobular stromal tissue, the ultrasound morphology is that of a hyperechoic enlargement of the TDLU

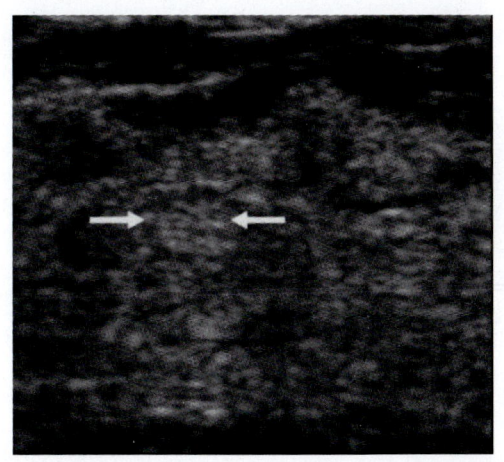

Fig. 11.3: In fibrocystic change when dilated TDLUs become distended with material they can present as uniformly echogenic solid lesions

Chapter 12

Evaluation of a Nipple Discharge

The availability of high resolution images from currently available equipment and the use of 11-gauge directional vacuum-assisted biopsy (DVAB) have greatly expanded the role of ultrasound in the evaluation and management of nipple discharge. Most patients with a nipple discharge have no palpable abnormality. Mammograms are normal in over half the patients with a nipple discharge even when a malignant pathology is the cause of the discharge. The usual investigation in these patients was X-Ray galactography but this is being increasingly supplanted by ultrasound as the primary investigative modality.

The causes of the discharge include Large Duct Papillomas (LDP), fibrocystic change (FCC), duct ectasia, carcinoma and a host of hyperplasias as well as hyperprolactinaemia. In any patient the cause may be multiple lesions.

HISTOLOGICAL BASIS OF IMAGE MORPHOLOGY

Intraductal papillomas (IDPs) are ductal proliferations around a fibrovascular core. Centrally located IDPs are also called large duct papillomas (LDPs). LDPs often contain adenosis, sclerosing adenosis, papillary apocrine metaplasia, varying degrees of hyperplasia and even carcinomas. Peripheral papillomas (PPs) arise in the TDLUs and are associated with epithelial proliferation including usual ductal hyperplasia (UDH), florid papillary hyperplasia (FDH/PDH), atypical duct hyperplasia (ADH) and ductal carcinoma in situ. Papillomatosis is the term used to describe multiple papillomas. Papillomas cause ductal dilatation and pour fluid into the ducts. They may undergo infarction and necrosis. Obstruction and secretion may cause the duct to form a cystic loculation: intracystic papillomas (ICPs).

Duct ectasia is a consequence of inflammation and dilatation consequent to autoimmune mechanisms or chronic hyperprolactinaemia. It evolves through the stages of dilatation and inflammation, cyst rupture, periductal mastitis and finally periductal fibrosis and hyperelastosis. The thick, pasty secretions within ectatic ducts are called comedomastitis.

Peripheral dilated TDLUs which contain papillary apocrine metaplasia are seen in fibrocystic change. These can cause an intermittent discharge which often coincides with the regression of the associated tender lump in the breast.

Ultrasound Morphology

The image morphology of papillomas (Figs 12.1 to 12.3) depends on the size, associated duct fluid, ductal expansion, ductal extension and peripheral or central location. The spectrum includes:
- Heterogeneous solid nodule with a thin, echogenic capsule and enhanced through transmission
- Microlobulated nodule

88 STEP BY STEP BREAST ULTRASOUND

- Intracystic nodule with or without duct extension
- Nodule with proximal and/or distal duct ectasia
- Branching or arborising ductal lesion.

The image morphology cannot differentiate between LDP, ADH or DCIS.

Ductal ectasia is well appreciated on ultrasound and is seen as variable combinations of:

- Dilated ducts with anechoic, hypoechoic or echogenic contents
- Absence of Doppler signals from the contents

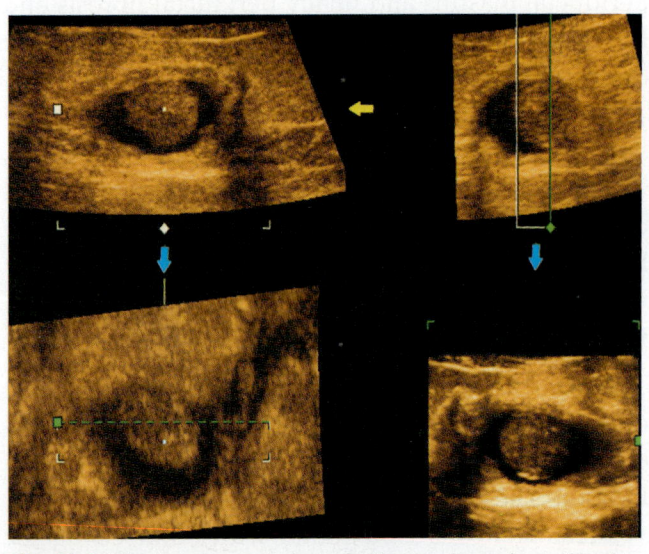

Fig. 12.1: The image morphology papillomas depends on the size associated ductal dilatation, ductal extension and duct fluid. This 3D reconstruction shows a homogeneous intracystic solid nodule within dilated fluid filled duct

EVALUATION OF A NIPPLE DISCHARGE 89

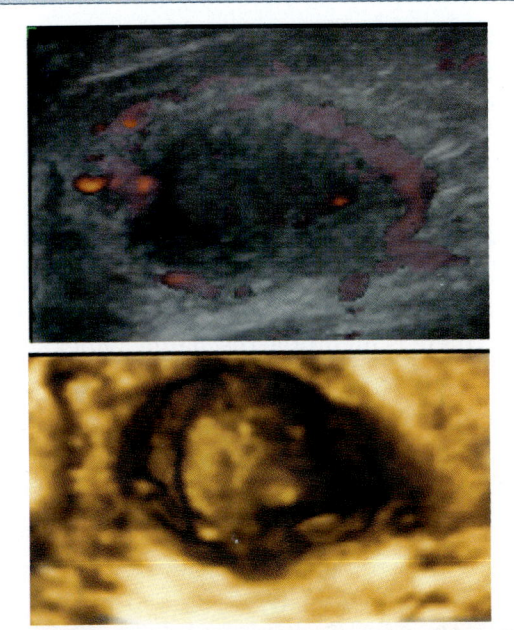

Fig. 12.2: This is a heterogeneous vascular intraductal papilloma. Image morphology does not differentiate between a large duct papilloma (LDP), atypical duct hyperplasia (ADH) and ductal carcinoma in situ (DCIS)

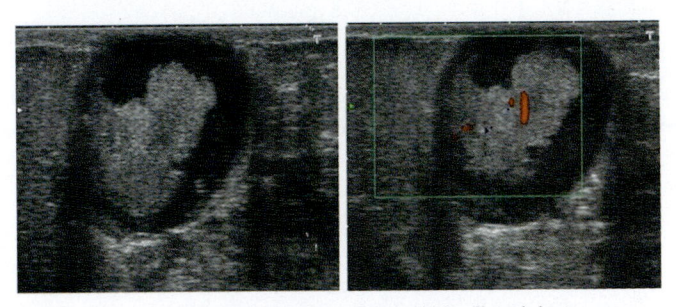

Fig. 12.3: Microlobulated nodules within dilated ducts may be benign or malignant

- Periductal oedema and wall thickening representing periductal mastitis
- Intraductal and periductal calcification.

FCC manifestations are similar to lesions not associated with a nipple discharge.

INTERVENTIONAL PROCEDURES

These include situations where galactography fails because there is no nipple discharge. Other situations include failure of cannulation of ducts, contrast extravasation and patient refusal. Ultrasound is useful for mammotomy guidance as well.

Chapter 13

Assessing the Breast Lump

In patients who have a palpable lesion and *have had a mammogram*, additional evaluation with ultrasound is useful:
- To confirm that the mammographic lesion coincides with the palpable lesion
- When the breast is dense or when the palpable lesion is in an area of dense breast tissue
- When the findings are non-specific
- When the findings are probably benign
- To confirm features of malignant disease and expedite a biopsy
- To prevent short-interval mammographic follow-up
- To determine the extent of malignant disease
- To guide interventional procedures
- When the palpable lesion is very superficial and therefore likely to be burned out with current techniques.

Increasingly, therefore, all palpable abnormalities are being evaluated with ultrasound as well, in spite of already having had a mammogram.

In patients who have a palpable abnormality and *have not had a mammogram*, ultrasound is useful:
- To demonstrate the structural equivalent of the abnormality
- To study perilesional tissues
- To guide interventional procedures.

Normal structures account for most lumps felt by the patient or the referring physician. The most *common ultrasound diagnoses* include:
- Echogenic interlobular fibrous stroma
- Simple cysts.
  Other diagnoses are also largely benign and include:
- Focal fibrosis
- Fibrous ridges
- Isoechoic glandular tissue
- Adenosis
- Fat lobules
- Costochondral junctions
- Fibroadenomas
- Carcinomas
- Lymph node.

Accuracy and *correlation can be enhanced* by:
- Fixing the lesion between index finger and middle finger
- Using a straightened clip in the field of view of the transducer or a worn out ball-point pen that can be kept on the lesion for correlation
- Asking the patient about a second or even a third or a fourth lesion that she is aware of, and examining that region as well.
- Palpating ridges from medial to lateral and lateral to medial aspect as well, as they are often asymmetric in their gradient
- Using a thick layer of gel or a stand-off pad to offset reverberation echoes in a near field lesion.

Chapter 14

Solid Lesions: Benign Versus Malignant

There is no way ultrasound can distinguish all benign solid lesions from all malignant lesions. This, however, does not mean that all solid lesions need to be biopsied. As in mammographic practice, ultrasound can offer the options of likely benign diagnosis and short-interval follow-up re-evaluation. This has been rendered possible consequent to the availability of high resolution equipment along with the acquisition of operator expertise.

As in mammography, the differentiation is based on the presence or absence of multiple features rather than depending on any one unique feature. It is important to keep in mind that standards have been defined to categorize differentiating features and that these should be adhered to strictly rather than loosely.

It is important to realise that breast cancer is not a single histopathologic entity and that various types exist. The imaging of breast cancer is further complicated by the fact that the pathologic basis of imaging depends not only on tumour tissue characteristics but on host responses to tumour tissue as well. Breast cancer is, therefore, heterogeneous and varies from nodule to nodule and even within a nodule.

The pathologic basis of image characterisation includes the following considerations:
- Desmoplasia which consists of fibrosis and elastosis is a host response to tumour. Spiculation of the

margins seen in ultrasound images (Figs 14.1 to 14.3) indicates that the tumour has given the host tissue time to respond and is therefore likely to be a slow growing, low to intermediate grade malignancy.
- Desmoplasia causes complete and partial acoustic shadowing (Fig. 14.4); cellular circumscribed lesions show enhanced through transmission (Fig. 14.5).
- Desmoplastic lesions are stiff and show up on elastography and display changes with vocal fremitus.
- Circumscribed cancers are high grade invasive ductal carcinomas that do not allow desmoplasia to

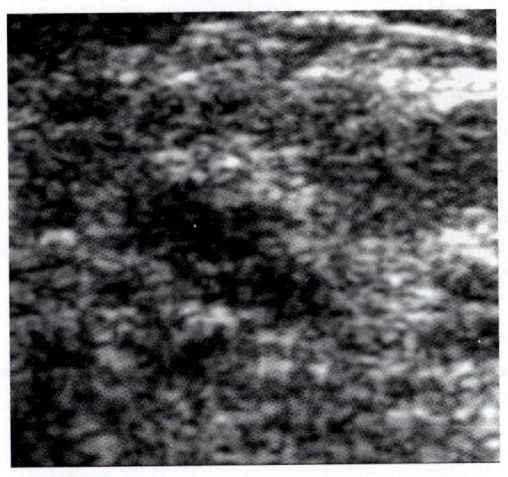

Fig. 14.1: Host tissue response to the presence of tumour tissue with fibrosis and elastosis. This constitutes desmoplasia and indicates that the host tissue has had time to respond. This is usually seen in low to intermediate grade malignancy and is evident as spiculation of the margins of the lesion

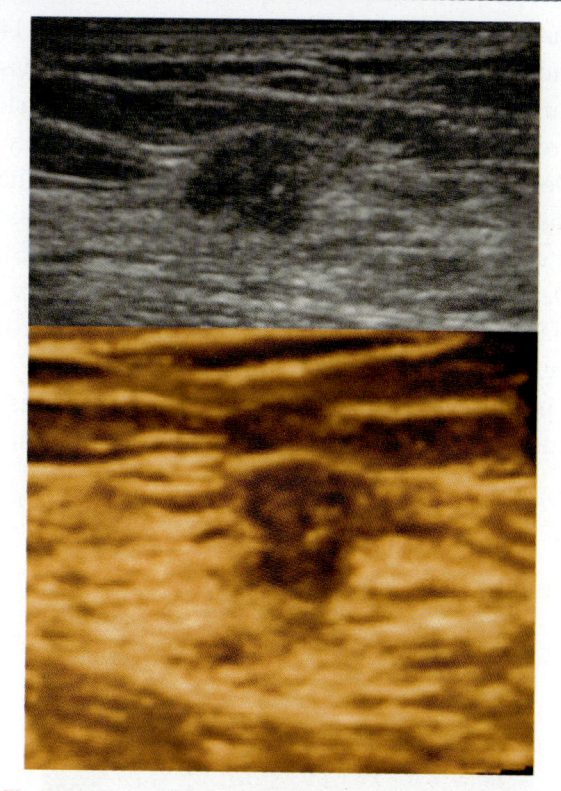

Fig. 14.2: Spiculation appears as a saw-toothed appearance of the outline of the lesion. The teeth can be shallow, deep, linear or curvilinear. The enhanced contrast resolution of three dimensional ultrasound techniques markedly increases the appreciation of spiculation

SOLID LESIONS: BENIGN VERSUS MALIGNANT

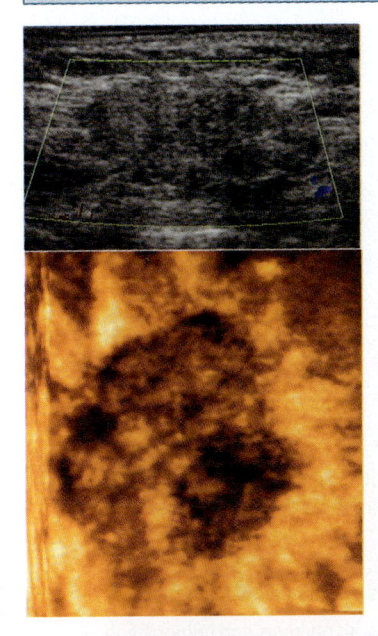

Fig. 14.3: This poorly delineated hypoechoic lesion shows excellent demonstration of a spiculated margin on a three dimensional reconstruction study

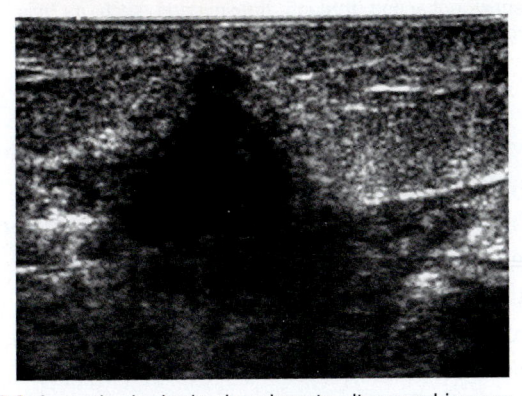

Fig. 14.4: Acoustic shadowing is unique to ultrasound images. It is an index of desmoplasia induced by malignant tumour tissue. This hypoechoic irregular lesion shows marked acoustic shadowing and was an invasive ductal carcinoma

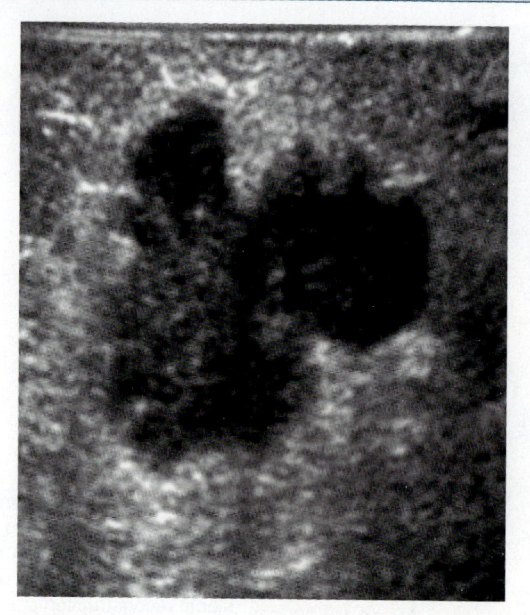

Fig. 14.5: Cellular lesions with necrosis and hemorrhage show enhanced through transmission such as this medullary carcinoma

develop. These tumours show a marked inflammatory response.
- Circumscribed lesions are more cellular and contain large numbers of tumour cells or lymphocytes or both.
- Circumscribed tumours are not stiff and may be missed on elastography.
- Circumscribed tumours are vascular (Fig. 14.6).

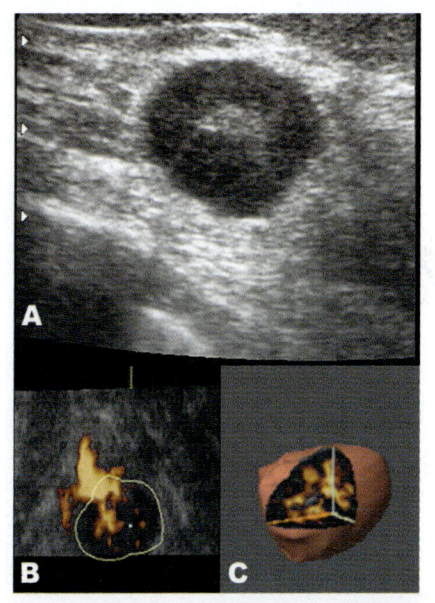

Fig. 14.6: Circumscribed malignant tumours (A) are cellular and contain large number of tumour cells and lymphocytes. These show extensive vascularity (B). Three dimensional power Doppler studies (C) are useful for quantifying tumour mass and displaying vascular morphology. Abnormal tumour morphology and subtle marginal discontinuity may sometimes be the only signs on ultrasound images of such lesions

- Lesions that show a combination of circumscribed and spiculated margins represent variable grade carcinomas with variable host response (Fig. 14.7).
- Spiculated tumours have few tumour cells and show little tumour vascularity (Fig. 14.8).
- Benign lobulations are large, gentle and few in number (Fig. 14.9). Microlobulations, which are a good marker for malignancy are smaller (1-2 mm), numerous and closer (Fig. 14.10).

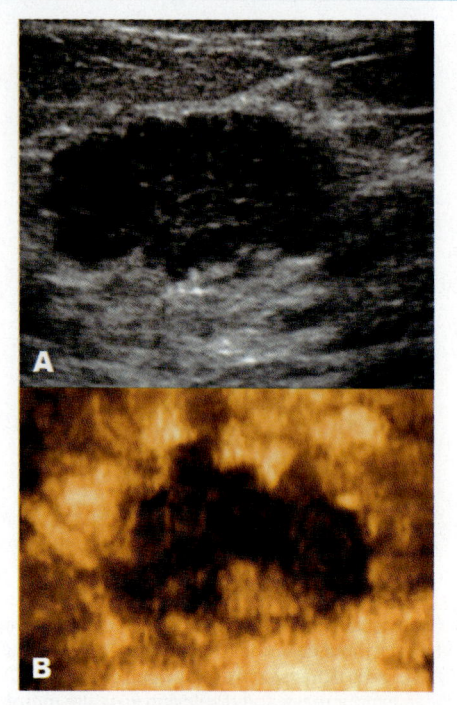

Fig. 14.7: Malignant tumours that have a variable cellular grade show a variable host response and a combination of circumscribed and spiculated margins (A). Three dimensional reconstruction (B) enhances visualisation of subtleties in the outline of a lesion

- Tumour invasion into the anterior mammary fascia and Cooper's ligaments, into periductal stromal tissue and into fat results in angular margins (Fig. 14.11) which is the most sensitive marker for malignancy. Angular margins are seen in both spiculated and circumscribed lesions.

SOLID LESIONS: BENIGN VERSUS MALIGNANT

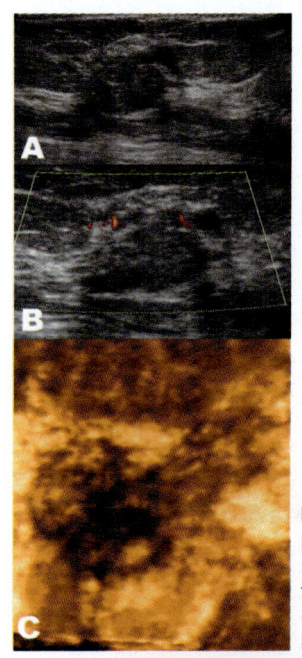

Fig. 14.8: Spiculated tumours have a poor cellularity (A) and show scanty tumour vascularity (B) even on very low flow power Doppler studies. 3D studies (C) show extensive spiculation in this largely avascular tumour

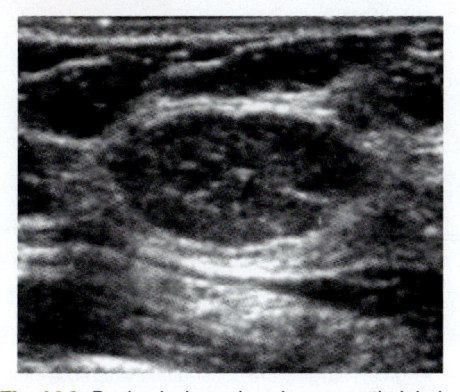

Fig. 14.9: Benign lesions show large, gentle lobulations that are a few in number. This is a gently lobulated fibroadenoma

104 STEP BY STEP BREAST ULTRASOUND

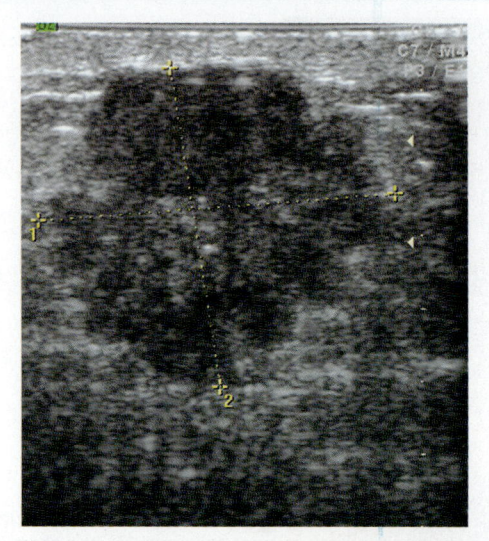

Fig. 14.10: Microlobulations are a good marker for malignancy. Compare to benign lesions these are smaller, closer and more numerous

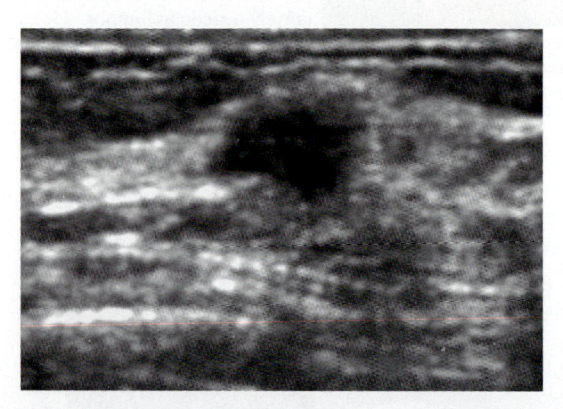

Fig. 14.11: Angular margins are consequent to tumour infiltration into periductal stromal tissue and this sign is one of the most sensitive markers for malignancy as in this invasive ductal carcinoma

SOLID LESIONS: BENIGN VERSUS MALIGNANT

- Malignant lesions become taller than wide (Fig. 14.12) as they grow. This is because of the general direction of terminal ductolobular units, because malignant tissues grow across tissue planes and because desmoplasia prevents them from getting compressed in an anteroposterior axis when transducer compression is applied.
- Both benign and malignant lesions show duct extension making it an unreliable single marker for malignancy.
- Calcification is a mammographic finding applied to ultrasound (Figs 14.13 to 14.15). Benign calcifications are often volume averaged. Many calcifications in the breast do not occlude the beam and are, therefore, not always associated with distal acoustic shadowing.

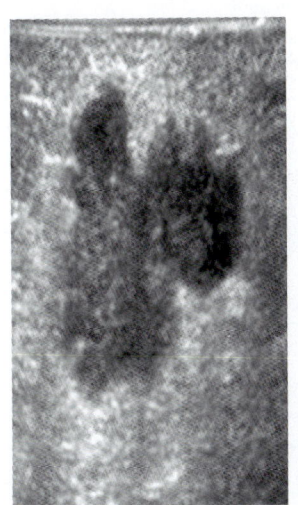

Fig. 14.12: Malignant lesions grow taller than wide. This is because of the general direction of most TDLUs and tumour invasion across tissue planes

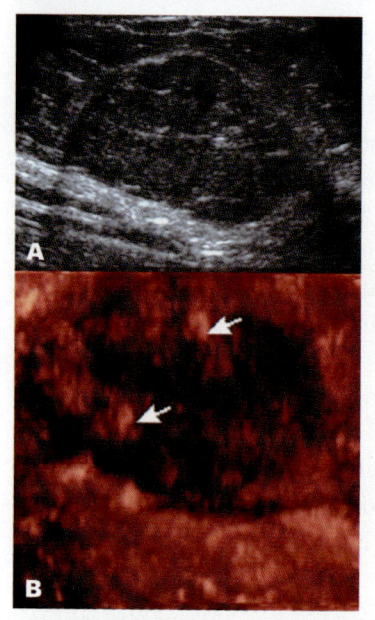

Fig. 14.13: Calcification in solid tumours is a mammographic findings applied to ultrasound. Sensitivity of ultrasound for calcification does not match that of mammography and calcific areas are usually identified during ultrasound only when they are specifically looked for (A). Three dimensional acquisitions (B) permit a study of the entire volume data set and therefore improve the sensitivity of ultrasound detection of calcification

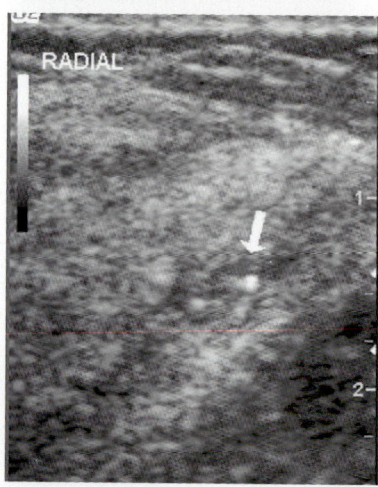

Fig. 14.14: Most calcifications do not occlude the ultrasound beam and are therefore not marked by distal acoustic shadowing

SOLID LESIONS: BENIGN VERSUS MALIGNANT

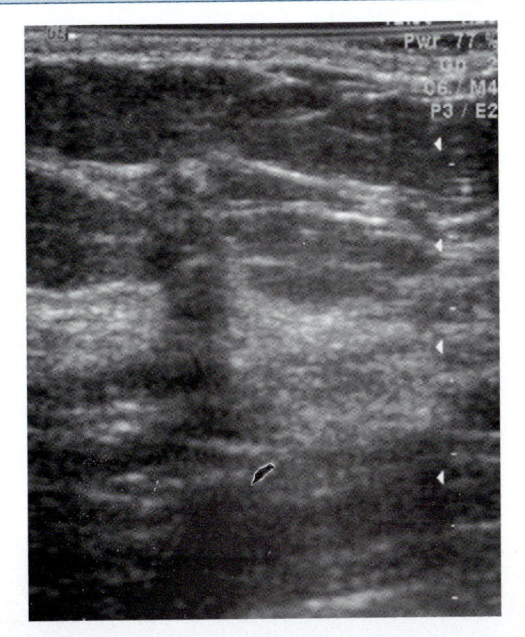

Fig. 14.15: When calcification is large and coarse enough, distal acoustic shadowing is evident

The relevance of using multiple image-morphology characteristics as markers for a malignant histopathologic diagnosis has been highlighted by Stavros and his group in recent published literature. Their findings are listed in Table 14.1.

Solid breast lesions that do not show any malignant stigmata should be assessed for benign features. These include:
- Purely hyperechoic tissue (Fig. 14.16)
- Elliptical and wider than tall shape (Fig. 14.17)

108 STEP BY STEP BREAST ULTRASOUND

Table 14.1: Sensitivities of individual and combined findings

Sonographic findings	Sensitivity
Microlobulations	92%
Angular margins	90%
Marked hypoechogenecity	49%
Duct extension	49%
Taller than wide	48%
Branch pattern	44%
Calcifications	40%
Spiculations	36%
Thick, echogenic halo	35%
Spiculations or thick halo	71%
Acoustic shadowing	35%
Combined sensitivity	99.6%

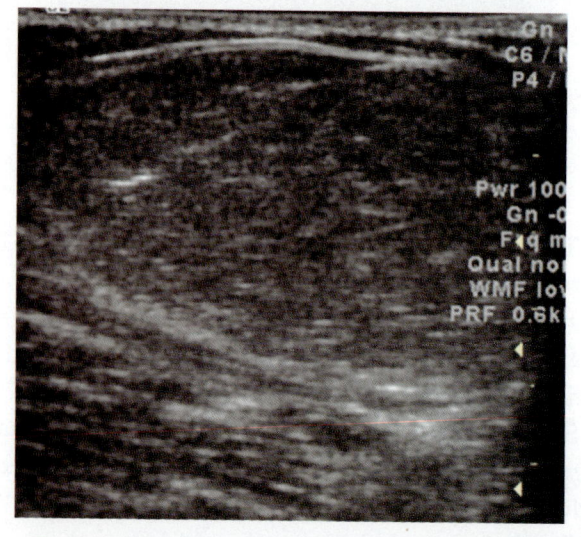

Fig. 14.16: Purely hyperechoic lesions are usually benign

SOLID LESIONS: BENIGN VERSUS MALIGNANT

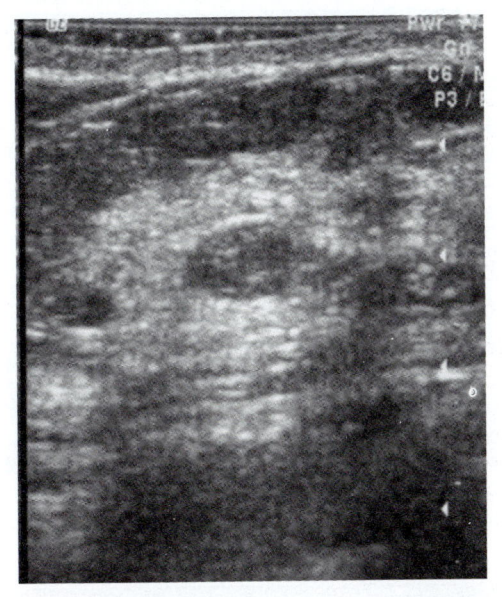

Fig. 14.17: Solid lesions that show no malignant features, are elliptical in shape and wider than tall almost always benign

- Gently lobulated and wider than tall shape (Fig. 14.18)
- A complete, thin, echogenic capsule (Fig. 14.19).

It should be remembered that although many circumscribed invasive carcinomas and most pure ductal carcinomas in situ have a complete, thin, echogenic capsule, they almost never have an elliptical or gently lobulated, wider than tall shape.

A useful algorithm for assessing lesions is as follows:
- Look for malignant characteristics; if present classify as ultrasound BIRADS 4a, 4b or 5 and biopsy

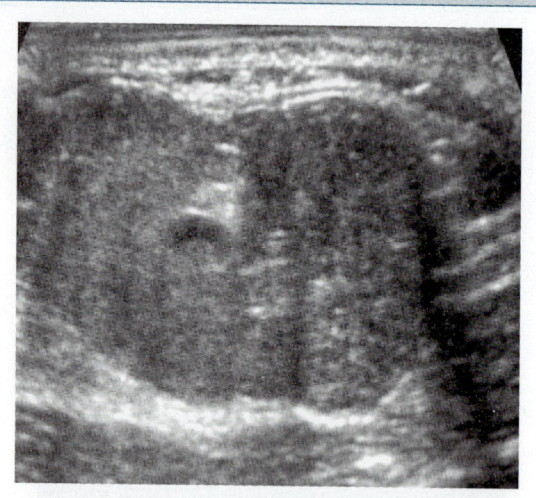

Fig. 14.18: Solid lesions that are wider than tall and gently lobulated are usually benign such as this fibroadenoma

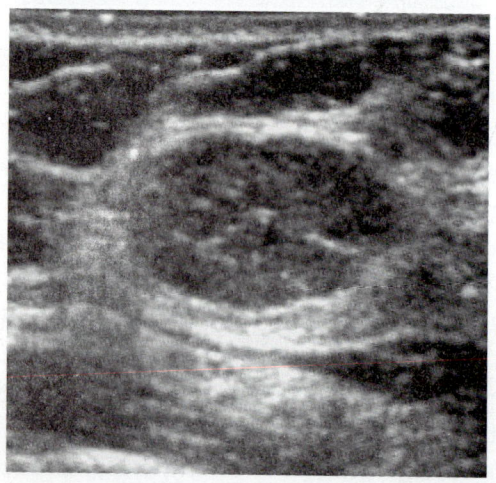

Fig. 14.19: When the capsule of a lesion is thin, complete and echogenic, the lesion is usually benign

SOLID LESIONS: BENIGN VERSUS MALIGNANT

- If malignant findings are not in evidence, look for benign findings; if present, classify as ultrasound BIRADS 2 or 3
- For BIRADS 3 offer three options: needle biopsy, surgical biopsy or follow-up
- If benign findings are not evident, classify as ultrasound BIRADS 4a and biopsy.

Characterising solid lesions into ultrasound BIRADS categories enhances the chances of identifying lesions missed on clinical examination or mammography. Equally important, it identifies lesions that do not require a biopsy when strict criteria are employed.

Specific features of some malignant lesions are as follows:

- Ductal Carcinoma In Situ (DCIS) is best assessed by mammography because mammography is more sensitive to identify and characterise microcalcifications. Most patients go straight from mammography to stereotactic biopsy. The role of ultrasound lies in those situations where a mammography shows a non-specific mass, for assessment of DCIS presenting as a nipple discharge and for needle localisation.
- Lobular Carcinoma In Situ is usually a biopsy diagnosis with no specific ultrasound findings. When it develops in a fibroadenoma or radial scar, the pre-existing lesion would be evident.
- Infiltrating duct carcinomas and breast carcinomas of no specific type show some or all of the features listed in Table 14.1.

- Medullary Carcinomas are markedly hypoechoic; show enhanced through transmission and show a nearly complete, thin echogenic capsule as a consequence of their pathological features of highly cellular growth, absence of desmoplasia, lymphoid infiltrates, necrosis and haemorrhage. A pseudocystic appearance similar to lymphomas may be apparent but the presence of internal vascular signals helps to exclude a cyst with echogenic debris or artefacts.
- Colloid carcinomas when small are isoechoic and difficult to identify. When larger than 15 mm, they have a salt and pepper appearance or are echogenic. They often have a thin echogenic capsule and enhanced through transmission without spiculation and can be mistaken for fat lobules, lipomas and fibroadenomas.
- Small tubular carcinomas are isoechoic, spiculated, have a thick echogenic halo and angular margins. Larger tubular carcinomas are hypoechoic, and cast prominent distal acoustic shadows.
- Intracystic papillary carcinomas need to be differentiated from fibrocystic lesions. Both may show thick walls, thick septations and mural nodules. When a nodule shows duct extension towards the nipple it should be considered malignant unless sampling proves otherwise.
- Invasive Lobular Carcinoma is often missed on mammography and not infrequently on ultrasound.

When seen, it manifests as any other malignant mass with multiple features. Ultrasound frequently underestimates the extent of the lesion.
- Non-Hodgkin's Lymphoma presents features of a cellular lesion with little or no desmoplasia.

Chapter 15

Solid Lesions: Specific Benign Diagnoses

Fibroadenomas

- Benign tumours that arise from the TDLU
- More common in a younger age group and oestrogen is thought to be responsible for formation and growth. Maximum incidence in the third decade; involute after menopause
- Contain variable amounts of stromal and epithelial elements and may undergo myxoid changes, sclerosis, hyalinization, calcification and infarction which can alter the echotexture
- Incorporate surrounding TDLUs that may then undergo proliferative and fibrocystic changes such as apocrine metaplasia, ductal hyperplasia, blunt duct adenosis, sclerosing adenosis; these are called complex fibroadenomas and these changes alter the echotexture. The presence of these changes in a fibroadenoma increases the relative risk for breast cancer development by 3.1-3.9. This translates to a 20% chance of developing a malignancy in the 25 years after the initial diagnosis of a complex fibroadenoma
- Usually have a pseudocapsule of compressed breast tissue. This is thin, complete and echogenic and is seen better with coded harmonics or Real-time compounding
- Usually no larger than 2 to 3 cm. Giant fibroadenomas may, however, grow rapidly and reach a size of upto 10 cm.

SOLID LESIONS: SPECIFIC BENIGN DIAGNOSES

- May rarely undergo malignant change (1 in 1000)
- Some phyllodes tumors arise in fibroadenoma
- Elliptical or gently lobulated in contour (Fig. 15.1); the more the lobulations and the smaller the size of the lobulations, the larger the risk of malignancy. Sclerosing adenosis makes the fibroadenoma margins appear angular and the lesion can then no longer be classified as benign
- Wider than tall orientation (Fig. 15.2)
- Most fibroadenomas are isoechoic or mildly hypoechoic compared to fat. Echogenecity depends

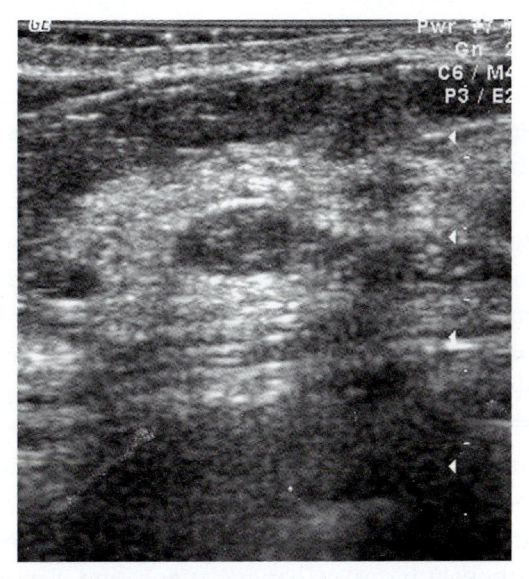

Fig. 15.1: The classical fibroadenoma is a homogeneously hypoechoic, wider than tall, mildly lobulated lesion with a thin echogenic capsule

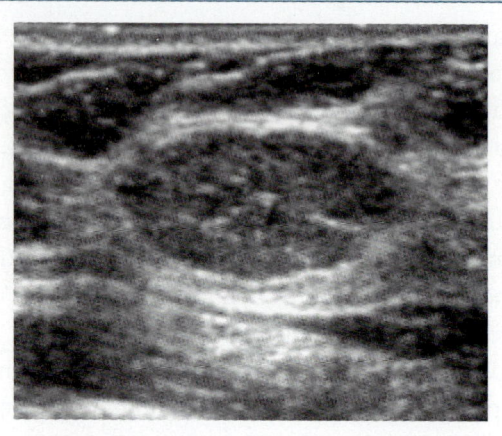

Fig. 15.2: Fibroadenomas are always wider than tall and may be isoechoic with surrounding fat

on cellular content, degenerative changes and transducer frequency. Epithelial elements result in a hypoechoic texture and stromal elements impart an isoechoic texture. A cellular stroma appears more hypoechoic and an acellular stroma appears more isoechoic. Sclerosis, hyalinisation and calcification tend to be hyperechoic (Fig. 15.3). Myxomatous changes are hypoechoic. Nodules that are completely isoechoic with a 5 MHz transducer appear relatively hypoechoic with a 7.5 MHz broad bandwidth transducer. Echogenecity is important to note because many benign-looking lesions on ultrasound are increasingly being followed up without a biopsy. Changes suggesting a complex fibroadenomas (Fig. 15.4) must be biopsied because

SOLID LESIONS: SPECIFIC BENIGN DIAGNOSES 119

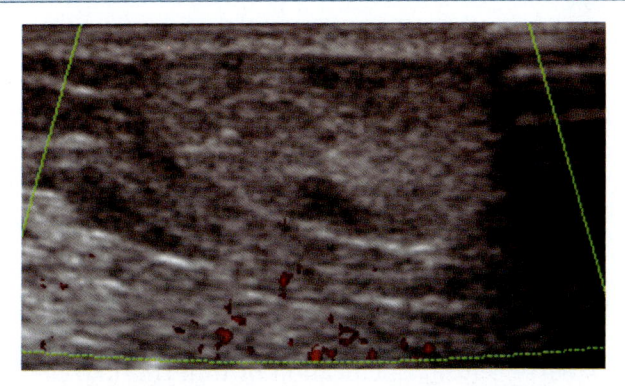

Fig. 15.3: When a fibroadenoma undergoes sclerosisor hyalinisation, its contents appear hyperechoic

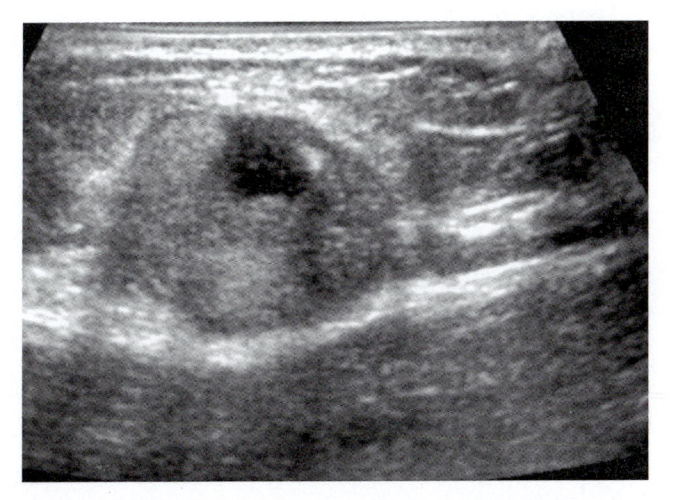

Fig. 15.4: Complex fibroadenomas show a heterogeneous echo pattern. These should lead to a mammographic surveillance at an earlier age

histologic evidence of a complex fibroadenoma leads to a mammographic surveillance at an earlier age. Many pathology departments do not differentiate between simple and complex fibroadenomas. This defeats the purpose of the biopsy as the aim is to identify a lesion that would need increased surveillance. It is, therefore, important to inform the pathologist that a complex fibroadenoma is being specifically looked for:

- Coarse central calcification or thin rim-like calcification may be evident
- Sound transmission is equal to or increased in comparison to surrounding tissues
- Usually mobile, unless infarcted
- Mildly compressible; the more the stromal component, the lesser the compressibility
- May be multiple and bilateral
- About half of all fibroadenomas have classis ultrasound features; the others should be histologically sampled
- Thin edge shadow
- Mobile
- Slightly compressible on transducer pressure

Tubular Adenomas/Lactating Adenomas

- Represent a single pathologic lesion in different stages of activity
- Consist of tubules indistinguishable from tubules in normal tissue. Lactating adenomas have true acini filled with secretions

SOLID LESIONS: SPECIFIC BENIGN DIAGNOSES

- Are indistinguishable from fibroadenomas on mammograms
- On ultrasound, tubular adenomas are wider than tall, hypoechoic and tend to be fusiform with variably pointed ends (Fig. 15.5); a minority are microlobulated and would need histologic sampling. Infarction can result in acoustic shadowing
- Lactating adenomas are hypoechoic, show enhanced through transmission, often have an incomplete thin surrounding capsule and are frequently microlobulated. Microlobulations are secondary to secretion distended acini and result in categorising the lesion as 4a.

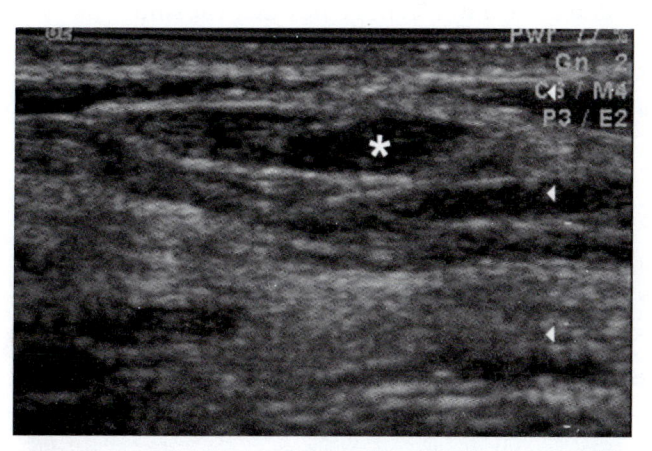

Fig. 15.5: Tubular adenomas are benign solid lesions, wider than tall, hypoechoic and fusiform. The ends are variably pointed

Intramammary Lymph Nodes

- Common finding on mammograms, often showing a classical fatty mediastinum which needs no further evaluation
- If the fatty hilum is not distinct on a mammogram, ultrasound shows an echogenic hilum
- Most frequent in the upper outer quadrants and in the tail; fairly frequent near the lateral margin of the sternum
- Have a normal echo pattern of a thin cortex and a bulky medulla (Fig. 15.6); pseudocystic appearance is a marker for metastatic deposits
- Normal lymph nodes are elliptical, markedly hypoechoic, less than 10 mm when intramammary and have a thin echogenic outer capsule

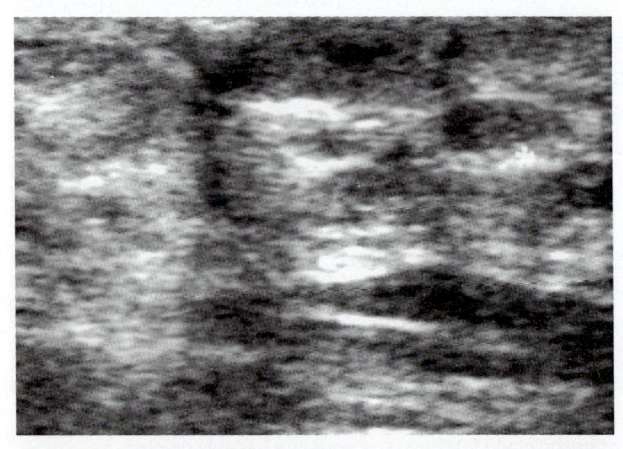

Fig. 15.6: Intramammary lymph nodes have the same echogenecity as lymph nodes elsewhere: an echogenic core surrounded by a hypoechoic rim

SOLID LESIONS: SPECIFIC BENIGN DIAGNOSES

- Malignant lymph node involvement renders them larger, rounder and alters the echotexture. Eccentric cortical thickening, rat-bite indentations of the cortex, severe eccentric mediastinal displacement or complete obliteration of the mediastinum favour a diagnosis of metastatic disease.

Hamartomas

- Unlike hamartomas elsewhere in the body, these likely represent fibrous and epithelial elements entrapped in a lipomatous growth
- Do not increase risk for malignancy
- Frequently asymptomatic and chance finding on mammograms
- Underdiagnosed histologically because they consist of variable amounts of normal fibrous, glandular and fatty elements
- May undergo apocrine metaplasia and cystic dilatation
- On mammography show a mixture of fat and water densities and may be round or oval; often the mammogram is conclusive without a biopsy
- Show a heterogeneous echotexture consequent to varying amounts isoechoic and tubular elements and echogenic fibrous tissue
- Smaller hamartomas lack a thin, echogenic capsule because this is actually a pseudocapsule of compressed tissue

- Compression reduces the lesion about one-third or so and makes it horizontally wider than tall shape.

LIPOMAS

- Benign overgrowths of adipose tissue
- Adipocytes are indistinguishable from normal breast fat adipocytes; the pathologist, therefore, needs to be informed about the fact that a mass suspicious of being a lipoma has been sampled
- May contain glandular tissue (adenolipomas) or capillaries (angiolipomas)
- Usually in the premammary zone; may lie in the mammary zone, pectoralis muscles or retropectoral space deep to muscle
- Not associated with increased relative risk of breast cancer development
- Mammography reveals a fat density with a water density pseudocapsule of varying thickness depending on size of lesion; may be obscured by water-density
- Classically benign lipomas, such as those with a mammographic BIRADS 2 appearance do not need an ultrasound
- Ultrasound is usually requested for assessing lumps seen on mammography as lesions lying in fibro-glandular tissue or for palpable lumps with negative mammographic findings
- Usually have an isoechoic echo pattern but may be more echogenic than surrounding fat (Fig. 15.7) and

SOLID LESIONS: SPECIFIC BENIGN DIAGNOSES 125

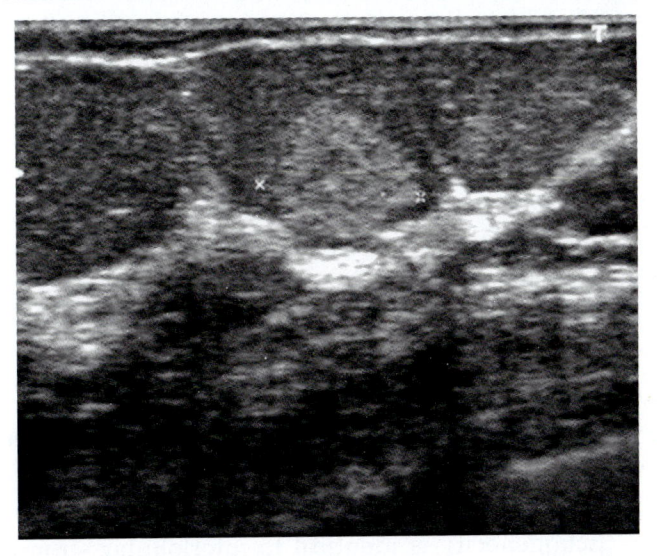

Fig. 15.7: Lipomas may be isoechoic or slightly more echogenic than surrounding fat. They appear as a fat density on mammography. An ultrasound is usually requested only for palpable lumps with negative findings

occasionally may have internal echogenic septa that course parallel to the skin
- Isoechoic lipomas that are slow growing and small may have an invisible pseudocapsule
- Normal fat lobules with or without necrosis may enlarge during rapid weight loss or weight gain

Focal Fibrosis

- Also known as fibrous mastopathy and chronic indurative mastitis

- Histologically consists of an area of largely acellular fibrous tissue containing occasional ductal and lobular elements that show no cystic dilatation
- No increased risk for cancer
- Usually in the upper, outer quadrants
- On mammograms appears usually as a tear-drop shaped opacity, variably circumscribed and with involutional calcification
- Ultrasound is usually done for either a palpable abnormality or a mammographic abnormality
- Appear as an intensely echogenic, homogeneous, biconvex or tear drop shaped, variably encapsulated nodule, wider than taller
- No central nidus is present
- Echogenecity is identical to interlobular stromal fibrous tissue

Diabetic Mastopathy

- Presents as a hard lump in premenopausal women with long-standing diabetes or as a mammographic abnormality
- Consists of collagenous stroma with abundant fibroblasts and B cell lymphocytes
- Self-limiting; but hardness always leads to biopsy
- Non-specific mammographic findings
- MRI with rotating delivery excitation off-resonance (RODEO) distinctively reveals no enhancement and is useful to differentiate it from invasive carcinoma
- No increased risk for cancer

SOLID LESIONS: SPECIFIC BENIGN DIAGNOSES

- Usually taller than wide, ill-defined, angular, microlobulated and with a central hypoechoic focus that has acoustic shadowing (Fig. 15.8); these features are remarkably similar to invasive ductal carcinoma, invasive lobular carcinoma and tubular carcinoma
- Are often bilateral and multifocal which is not reassuring, because invasive lobular carcinomas is also bilateral and multifocal

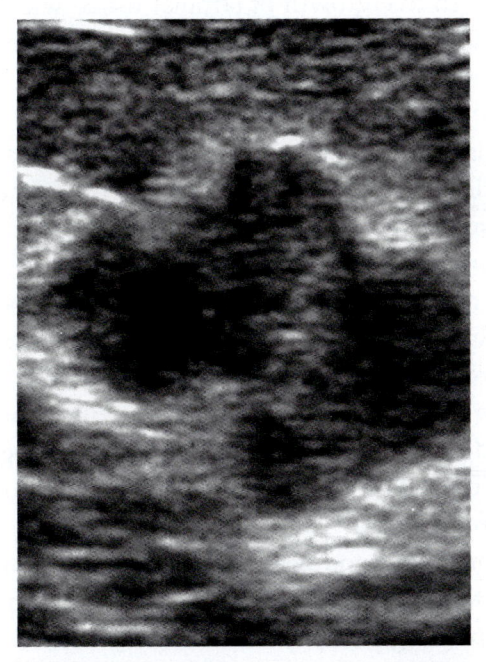

Fig. 15.8: Diabetic mastopathy presents as a taller than wide, poorly marginated or microlobulated lesion with variable acoustic shadowing. The hardness of these lumps usually leads to their biopsy

- Multifocal lesions may be synchronous or come up later while the patient is on follow-up
- Doppler may be helpful because diabetic mastopathy is avascular; this distinction is facilitated by the use of ultrasound contrast media which enhances vascularity of malignant lesions.

PSEUDOANGIOMATOUS STROMAL HYPERPLASIA (PASH)

- Benign overgrowth of stromal tissue which histologically consists of abnormally prominent stroma between lobules and ducts
- The stroma shows slit-like spaces which do not consist of intima-lined spaces containing red blood cells; these spaces contain disrupted collagen mucopolysaccharide and are lined with epithelial or myoepithelial cells (pseudoangiomas)
- Mammography shows them as circumscribed, non-calcified isodense lesions indistinguishable from fibroadenomas
- Ultrasound reveals a well-circumscribed, taller than wide, mildly hypoechoic, slightly heterogeneous lesion with a thin echogenic capsule, similar to a fibroadenoma
- Some PASH nodules may contain cysts. Some may be taller than wide, angular and microlobulated mandating a biopsy
- Hyperplastic stroma is avascular on colour Doppler and this helps to differentiate it from phyllodes tumours and cellular fibroadenomas

Granular Cell Tumours

- Also known as myoblastomas and have an origin in Schwann's cell
- Present as a mammographic or palpable abnormality
- May be associated with dimpling of overlying skin
- Usually located in the upper inner quadrants
- Are not premalignant
- Consist of sheets of spindle shaped cells with eosinophilic granules; some might show infiltrating margins which can masquerade as infiltrating scirrhous breast carcinomas
- Appear on mammograms as malignant nodules with spiculated, infiltrating margins; no calcification is evident
- Ultrasound findings are non-specific: an elliptical or fusiform nodule without a thin echogenic capsule
- Have a unique anisotropic effect. The lesion will appear hypoechoic when the beam strikes it at an oblique angle and mildly hyperechoic when the beam is nearly perpendicular to the internal fibrils. Commonly seen in tendons and not reported in any other breast lesion
- Some lesions show infiltrating margins and acoustic shadowing

Hemangiomas

- Usually clinically inapparent and also not visible on mammograms
- Microscopic perilobular hemangiomas are usually less than 4 mm across and are incidental histology findings
- Most macroscopic hemangiomas lie in the subcutaneous tissue and are truly skin lesions
- Hemangiomas may be capillary, cavernous or mixed types
- Are not reported in literature because they are too small
- Are variably echoic and may show punctate calcification representing phleboliths or thrombosis.

Fibrocystic Changes and Benign Proliferative Disorders

These are discussed in Chapter 12.

Chapter 16

High Risk and Premalignant Diagnoses

Some breast lesions have a marked propensity for a malignant change. These include:
- Atypical ductal hyperplasia
- Atypical lobular hyperplasia
- Phyllodes tumour
- Juvenile papillomatosis
- Radial scars
- Sclerosing papillomatosis.

These changes are not necessarily lesions that have a high propensity for malignant change within the lesion. Several of these are lesions that when present are associated with a synchronous malignant lesion in the same or contralateral breast. Additionally, some of these lesions show high local recurrence rates and can often show histopathologic features that are difficult to label as clearly benign or frankly malignant.

HYPERPLASIA

Common proliferative disorders of breast tissue include lobular hyperplasia, ductal hyperplasia and apocrine metaplasia with hyperplasia. Lobular and ductal varieties of hyperplasia have benign, atypical and intermediate forms.

Ductal hyperplasia refers to proliferation of the epithelial and myoepithelial layers of ducts within lobules and the terminal duct as well. There is a spectrum of this condition extending from benign to malignant. Usual Ductal Hyperplasia (UDH) is three to four cell layers thick. When the layers are five or more this is referred to as moderate UDH. When the hyperplasia tends to form into papillae and fills up and distends the ducts and acini it is called florid or papillary duct hyperplasia (PDH). When papillae develop a vascular core they are indistinguishable from papillomas. As proliferation progresses, the cells show less variability and uniform hyperchromatic nuclei and this pattern is referred to as Atypical Ductal Hyperplasia (ADH). These cells fill up and variably distend acini similar to Ductal Carcinoma In Situ (DCIS). Dystrophic calcification may be in evidence at this stage. DCIS and invasive duct carcinoma reflect the malignant end of the ductal hyperplasia spectrum. The increased risk for cancer in ADH is not necessarily in the area of ADH bit anywhere in the same breast and in the contralateral breast as well. The risk for cancer is twofold for mild UDH, threefold for moderate UDH, four to fivefold for ADH and eight to tenfold for ADH with a positive family history. The ultrasound features of ADH are those of the underlying lesion in which ADH develops (Fig. 16.1): enlarged TDLUs, enlarged terminal duct, Radial scar, fluid-filled central duct or a solidly full central duct and calcification. Not infrequently ADH is seen as a solid nodule with one or more suspicious markers: duct extension, a thick echogenic halo, microlobulation or spiculation. Fortunately most of these result in an ultrasound BIRADS 4 categorisation and therefore histological sampling.

Lobular hyperplasia refers to the pattern of hyperplasia and not its location and has a spectrum from benign lobular hyperplasia (BLH) to atypical lobular

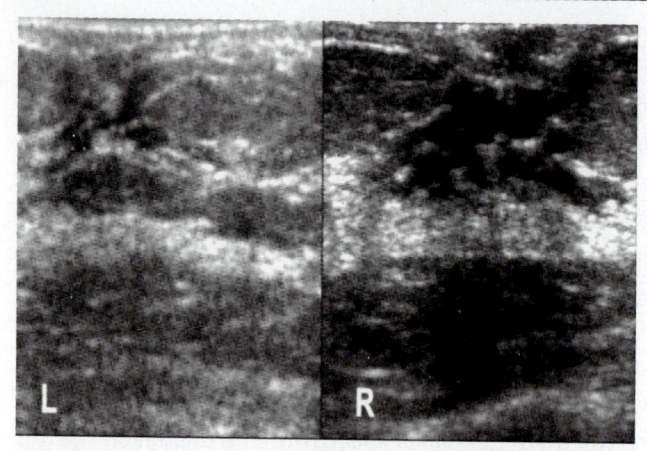

Fig. 16.1: Comparison of retroareolar ducts in the left and right breast of the same patient. There is an asymmetric enlargement of central ducts on the right side with variably echogenic contents and occasional calcification

hyperplasia (ALH) and Lobular Carcinoma In Situ (LCIS). ALH is a premalignant condition as well as a marker for an increased risk of cancer in the same or contralateral breast. It is often a coincidental lesion in a biopsy for a mammographic lesion or a palpable abnormality. Ultrasound findings include an isolated enlarged TDLU or the underlying lesion for which a biopsy was performed. These include adenosis, sclerosing adenosis, PDH, papillary apocrine metaplasia or a complex fibroadenoma.

JUVENILE PAPILLOMATOSIS

This is a controversial lesion. Some workers believe that the cancer risk associated with it is only that of associated ADH. Others believe its presence is premalignant or a general marker for cancer in either breast. Histologically the lesion consists of fibrocystic and proliferative changes. The proliferative changes include duct hyperplasia, usually florid or papillary. Ultrasound findings have scant reports in literature and include a solid lesion with peripheral cysts.

RADIAL SCARS AND SCLEROSING PAPILLOMATOSIS

Radial scars and sclerosing papillomatosis consist of a central fibrous core surrounded by proliferating ducts and lobules and fibrocystic changes. The cause is unknown and their significance lies in their resemblance to spiculated carcinomas on mammography. The role of ultrasound is minimal since these are usually mammographic lesions and are usually assessed by additional mammographic views or a mammographically directed stereotactic biopsy. Ultrasound is useful for preoperative localisation. Ultrasound findings are non-specific and depend on the extent of peripheral proliferative changes.

Phyllodes Tumour

Originally labelled Cystosarcoma Phyllodes, this tumour has been renamed Phyllodes tumour to indicate that it is not always malignant. About two-thirds of these are benign and one-third malignant. Some of the benign ones are locally recurrent.

Clinically these are rapidly growing masses that are picked up by palpation. One-fifth present as non-palpable mammographic screen findings. Prominent vein lie in the skin over the lesion. Internal cystic necrosis, haemorrhage and skin ulceration are not unusual. Histologically, the tumour consists of cellular stromal proliferation and epithelial elements and may arise in a fibroadenoma.

On mammography these usually appear as a large water density lesion with variable amounts of spiculation. Lesions larger than 30 mm across are more likely to be malignant.

Most Phyllodes tumours are solid nodules with a smooth echogenic thin capsule, occasional calcification, good through transmission and distal acoustic shadowing (Fig. 16.2). Cystic areas are common and may be round or classically flattened and also often appear as

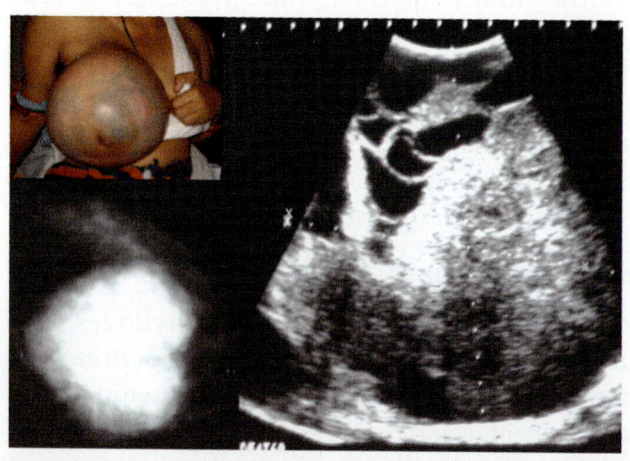

Fig. 16.2: Cystosarcoma Phyllodes is a rapidly growing breast mass that is not always malignant. On mammography these appeared as large water density lesions. On ultrasound these appear as a solid nodule but may also appear as a multiseptated fluid lesion. Even benign lesions are locally recurrent

horizontally oriented echogenic stripes. Malignant Phyllodes tumours are large, spiculated, incompletely marginated and often with angular margins. Some benign lesions are indistinguishable from fibroadenomas.

Chapter 17

Cystic Lesions

Breast cysts can be adequately evaluated by ultrasound alone and do not need a biopsy if they meet strict criteria. Complex cystic lesions, unlike as in other organs such as the liver or kidney, on the other hand, are usually benign but owing to their morphology, more frequently need a sampling to exclude a malignant neoplastic diagnosis.

Breast cysts are thin walled, fluid-filled spaces which may present as a lump, as nodularity, as a breast pain or as a chance imaging finding. These are hormone dependant and show cyclical changes. These may rupture or atrophy and disappear completely. They are more common in the upper outer quadrants.

The criteria for a simple cyst (Fig. 17.1) are:
- A completely anechoic area
- Well-circumscribed
- A complete, thin, echogenic capsule
- Enhanced through transmission
- Thin edge shadows.

Additional features that suggest a benign simple cyst include:
- Clusters of simple cysts (Fig. 17.2)
- Thin septations (Fig. 17.3)
- Milk of Calcium
- Punctate calcification in wall (Fig. 17.4)
- Eggshell calcification (Fig. 17.5).

CYSTIC LESIONS 141

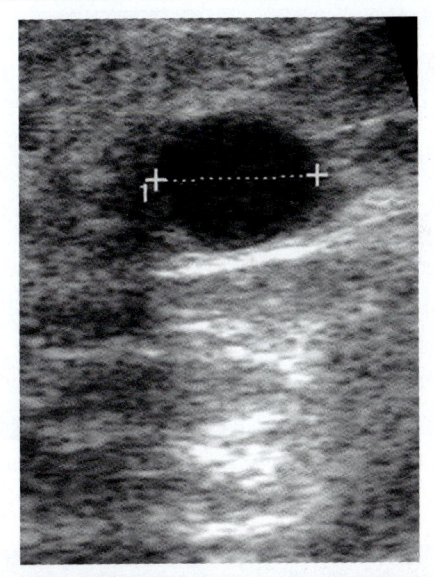

Fig. 17.1: The criteria for a simple cyst include a completely anechoic area which is well circumscribed, has a complete thin echogenic capsule and shows enhanced through transmission with thin edge shadows

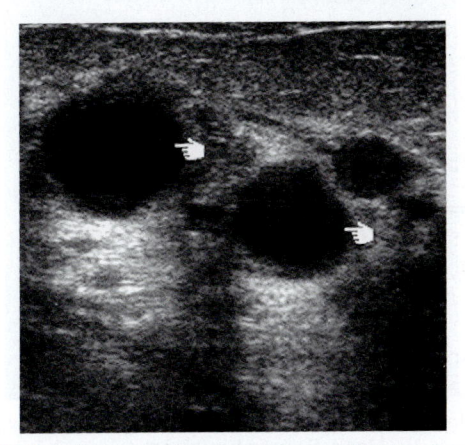

Fig. 17.2: A cluster simple cyst reinforces a benign diagnosis

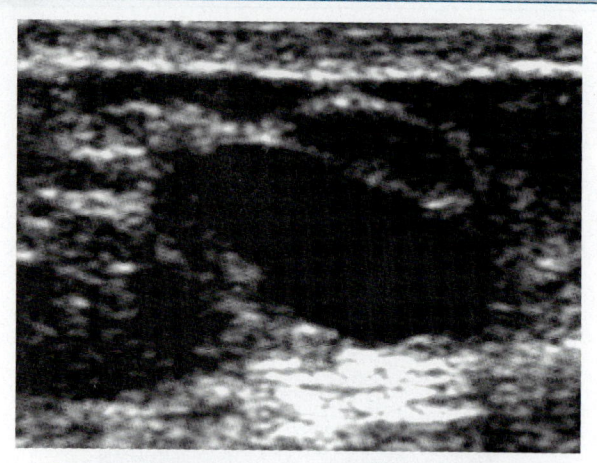

Fig. 17.3: Thin avascular septations in a cyst indicates cysts of a benign origin

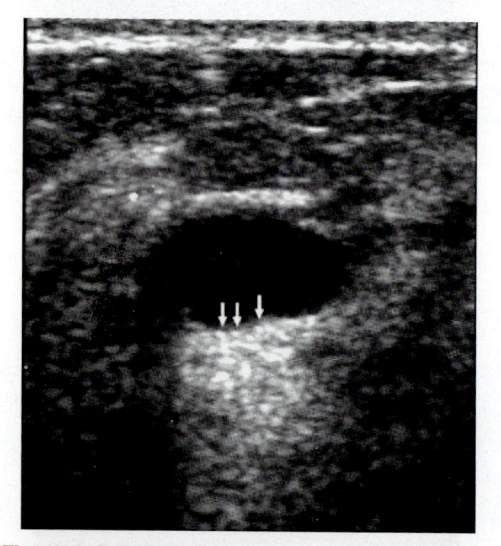

Fig. 17.4: Punctate calcification in a cyst wall is highly indicative of a benign aetiology

CYSTIC LESIONS

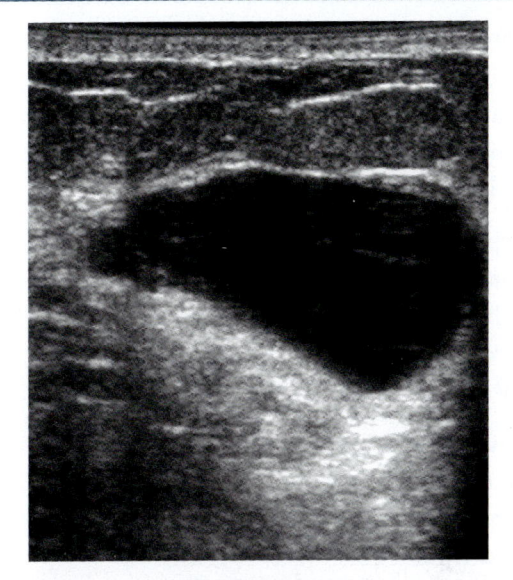

Fig. 17.5: Eggshell calcification in a cyst suggests a benign origin

Simple cysts rarely develop malignancy but may be invaded by an adjacent neoplasm.

Complex cysts are those cysts that do not meet the criteria for simple cysts.

Technical artefacts that can cause internal echoes include reverberation echoes, ring down pseudolesions, clutter, triangulation, speckle and side-lobe artefacts.

Causes of internal echoes in a cystic lesion include:
- Cellular debris
- Red blood cells, White blood cells and plasma cells
- Macrophages

- Protein globules
- Cholesterol crystals
- Floating or papillary epithelial cells
- Apocrine cells
- Papilloma/Carcinoma.

Suspicious findings in a breast cyst include:
- Mural nodules
- Multifrond, microlobulated contour
- Fibrovascular stalk
- Thick septations.

Signs of an inflammation in a cyst include:
- Circumferential wall thickening
- Hyperemia in the capsule
- Fluid-fluid levels.

Chapter 18

Complex Cystic Lesions

Some common conditions of the breast present as echogenic cystic lesions and may actually have phases appearing completely solid. These include:
- Galactoceles
- Mastitis and abscesses
- Fat necrosis
- Seromas, haematomas and lymphoceles
- Mondor's disease
- Hemangiomas, venous malformations and lymphangiomas

These lesions are largely inflammatory and their imaging findings overlap. The clinical perspective is, therefore, important to come to a final differential diagnosis.

Equally importantly, these conditions not infrequently evolve from one to another. Examples include haematomas and fat necrosis evolving into seromas or abscesses, galactoceles becoming infected and forming abscesses, and lumpectomy sites becoming fat necrosis.

A knowledge of these lesions is important in assessing the finer aspects of histopathologic possibilities based on ultrasound image characteristics and not expressing amazement at the final histopathology report!

Galactoceles

- Consist of terminal ducts, terminal ductules or TDLUs dilated with milk

COMPLEX CYSTIC LESIONS

- Usually present as painless lumps after cessation of breastfeeding
- May appear in pregnancy and during lactation as well
- Image morphology varies with status of contained fat droplets and with location
- Acute galactoceles contain well emulsified fat and appear anechoic (Fig. 18.1)
- Occasionally, numerous very fine low level mobile echoes are evident

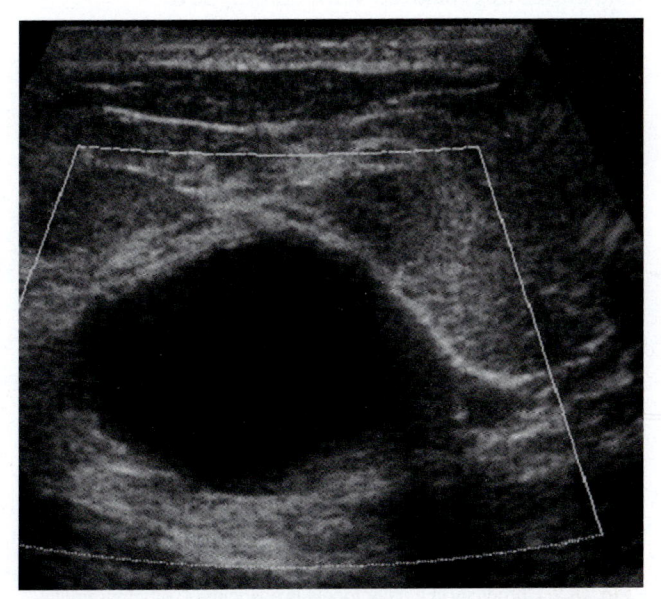

Fig. 18.1: Acute galactoceles contain fat which is largely well emulsified and therefore gives them a largely anechoic pattern

- Peripheral galactoceles are usually multilocular
- Central galactoceles are usually unilocular or bilocular
- Subacute galactoceles show uniform low levels echoes (Fig. 18.2)
- Old galactoceles are inhomogeneously echogenic or are homogeneously echogenic
- Colour flow may demonstrate flow in septa but not in the centre of the lesion in galactoceles differentiating them from malignant solid lesions
- Contained milk may swirl when disturbed and this is better appreciated with colour flow

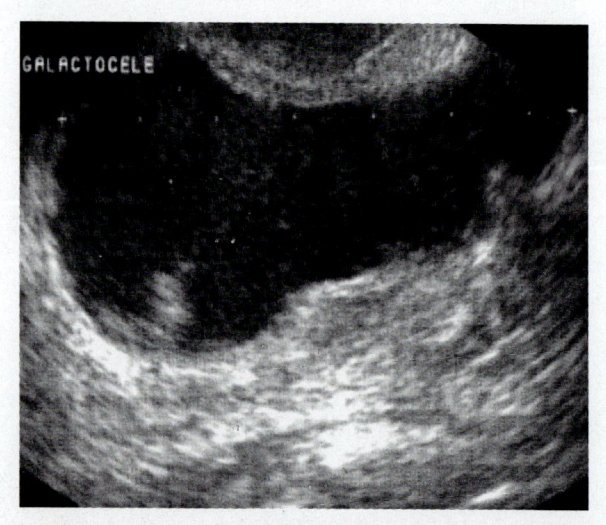

Fig. 18.2: Chronicity in a galactocele is associated with non-emulsified fat and inflammatory debris. This causes low level echoes

COMPLEX CYSTIC LESIONS 149

- May contain a fat-fluid level
- When findings are not conclusive an aspiration helps in diagnosis and may even be therapeutic.

Lactational Mastitis and Abscesses

- Nipple fissures, obstruction and stasis contribute to the inflammatory process in the lactating patient
- *Staphylococcus aureus* is the most common organism
- The onset is marked by acuteness and local and systemic signs of inflammation and sepsis
- Ultrasound is the investigation of choice
- Mammograms are either dense (due to lactation) or non-specific
- Ultrasound is used to detect an abscess as early as possible, to obtain a sample for Gram's staining, culture and sensitivity and to guide drainage
- Thickening and oedema result in decreased beam penetration (Fig.18.3) and a 5 Mz transducer actually has a better sensitivity than higher frequency transducers
- Ultrasound morphology depends on the duration and severity of the inflammatory process
- Split screen images of anatomically symmetric parts of the contralateral breast are very useful for comparison

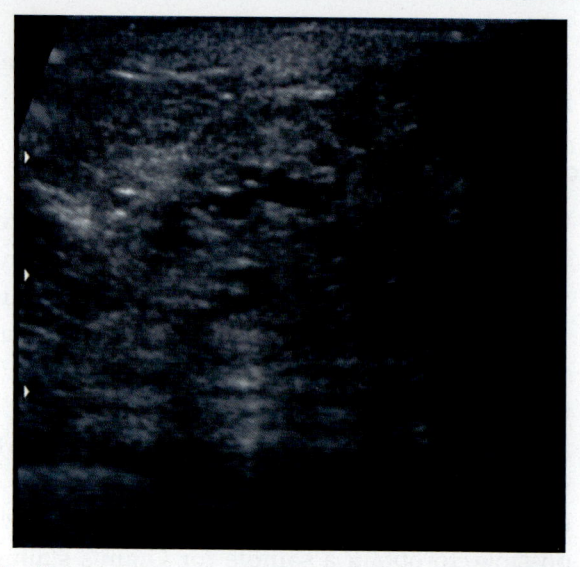

Fig. 18.3: Thickening and oedema as a consequence of mastitis appear as poorly marginated inhomogeneously hypoechoic areas which show markedly poor beam penetration

- Oedema is the earliest sign and is seen as an echogenic thickening of subcutaneous fat. Affected Cooper's ligaments and stroma become enlarged and hypoechoic (Fig. 18.4)
- As inflammation advances, textural changes between fat, stroma and ductules gets obscured (Fig. 18.5)
- Liquefaction results in abscess formation. This appears as a thick wall with variably echogenic material within (Fig. 18.6)

COMPLEX CYSTIC LESIONS

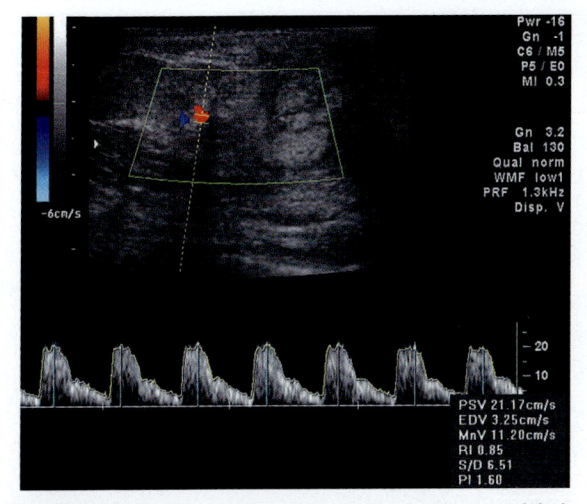

Fig. 18.4: As mastitis gets localised, it shows up as a globular area of increased or decreased echogenecity without a capsule and with variable hyperemia

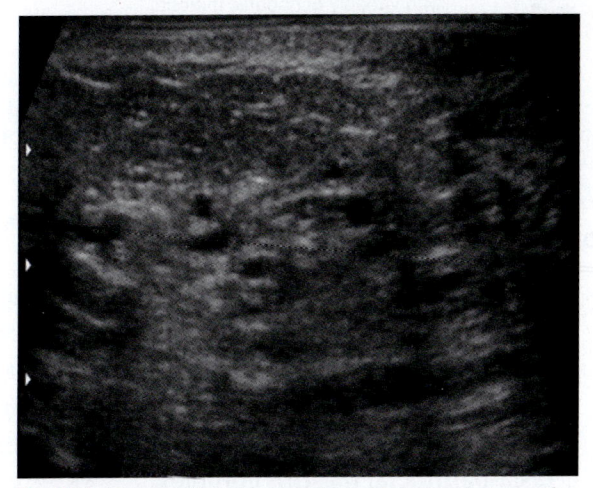

Fig. 18.5: Inflammation obscures textural changes between fat, stroma and ductules

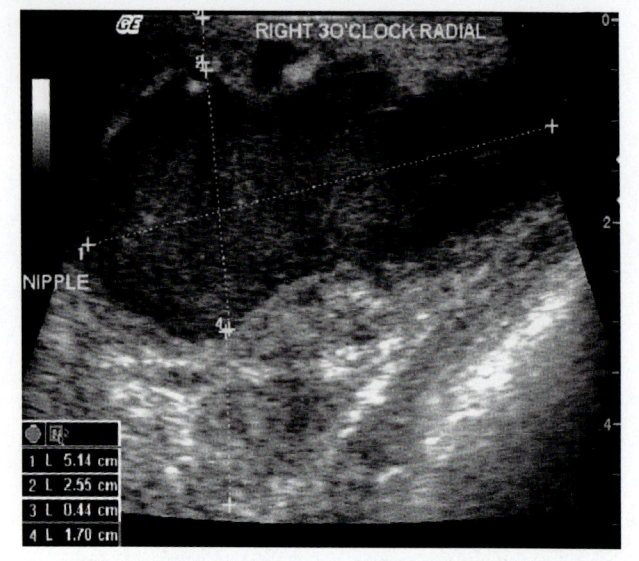

Fig. 18.6: Abscess formation appears as a thick wall with variably echogenic material

- Abscesses may be single or multiple
- Ultrasound guided drainage is emerging as a procedure of choice to treat abscesses.

Non-puerperal Mastitis and Abscesses

- May be bacterial or purely chemical inflammation
- Anaerobes are more frequent organisms
- Associated with duct ectasia very frequently; rupture and chemical inflammation are the usual sequence and hence the condition is called duct ectasia-periductal mastitis complex

COMPLEX CYSTIC LESIONS

- Predisposing factors include nipple inversion with associated squamous metaplasia in younger women and a hormonal basis in perimenopausal women
- Very likely multifactorial including diabetes mellitus, immunosuppressed states and intake of corticosteroid medication
- Mammographic findings are non-specific
- Ultrasound findings specifically include dilated subareolar ducts filled with variably echogenic fluid (Fig. 18.7)

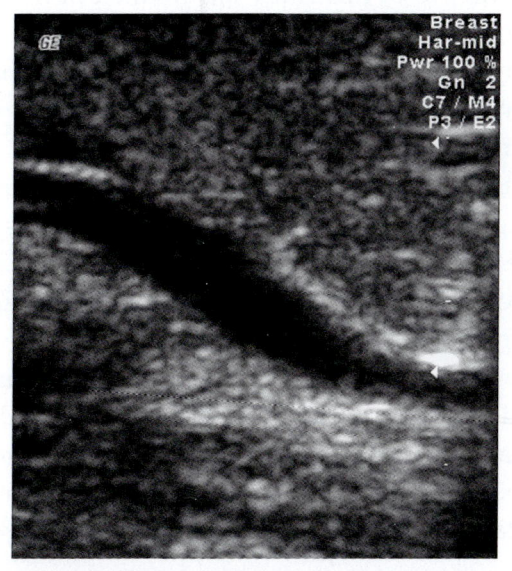

Fig. 18.7: Non-lactational abscesses show varied alterations of echogenecity in the subareolar region and specifically dilated subareolar ducts with variably echogenic fluid

- Other findings include oedema and an abscess cavity; the cavity is usually periareolar
- Colour flow and power Doppler may show hyperemia of the duct wall
- Chronic foci can present as solid nodules, intraductal calcification or periductal fibrosis
- Peripherally located foci of mastitis are usually secondary to fibrocystic change (FCC).

Tubercular Mastitis

- Awareness of this entity has resulted in increased diagnosis in recent times
- May present as a palpable abnormality, a mammographic finding, systemic symptoms or an inflammatory breast lesion
- Classical ultrasound signs include a lesion commencing in the fat or glandular tissue that extends up to the skin (Figs 18.8 to 18.10). This consists of finely irregular, hypoechoic spaces that coalesce as hypoechoic channels. Vascularity is minimal
- Non-specific changes are seen in early manifestations of the disease and include focal ductal dilatation with calcification and echogenic contents, a poorly marginated hypoechoic area or an area of focal oedema in fat or stroma.

COMPLEX CYSTIC LESIONS 155

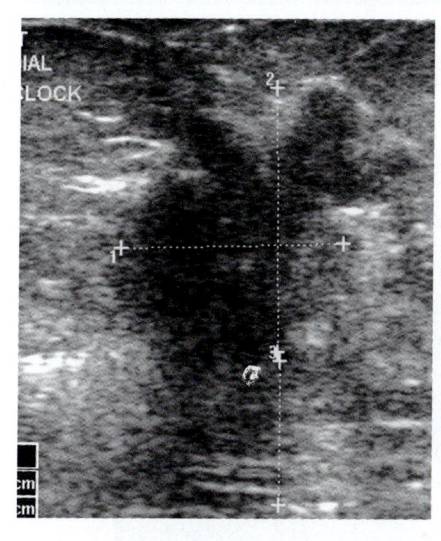

Fig. 18.8: Tubercular lesions in the breast are common in patients of asian origin. These appear as hypoechoic spaces with a finely irregular outline that coalesce as hypoechoic channels making their way towards the skin and not following anatomical axes

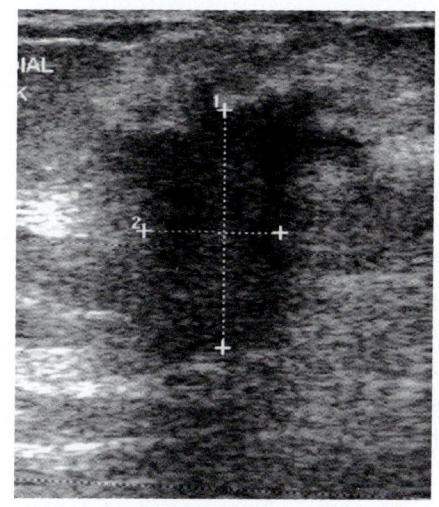

Fig. 18.9: This taller than wide lesion with spiculated margins and a hypoechoic pattern with minimal vascularity yielded caseating tubercular granulomas on a core biopsy

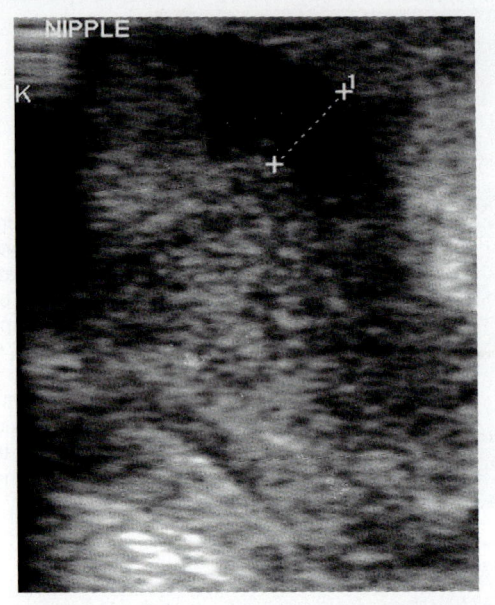

Fig. 18.10: Irregular hypoechoic lesion defying anatomical axes extending from the glandular elements to the nipple. A vacuum assisted biopsy yielded necrotic material and no tissue core. Staining and microscopy showed caseating granulomas

Seromas and Lymphoceles

- Localised collections of serous fluid
- May get secondarily infected
- Consequent to interventional procedures, surgical procedures or implant complications
- Internal echoes are due to fibrinous adhesions, blood, pus or lymph; pseudoseptations may be evident consequent to fibrinous coagulum
- Often have the shape of the original surgical defect.

Haematomas

- Usually consequent to a procedure; occasionally after injury or haemorrhage into a cyst
- Appearance varies with age; immediate appearances are of an anechoic structure; later the lesion evolves through a heterogeneously hypoechoic (fibrinous) to a hyperechoic (clot) phase and then onto nodules or fluid-fluid levels
- Chronic haematomas show enhanced through transmission and variably echogenic walls
- May be unilocular or multilocular
- Internal echoes are always avascular on colour flow and power Doppler studies.

Fat Necrosis

- Consequent to trauma, surgical intervention, ischemia of any cause, cyst rupture, ectatic duct rupture or haemorrhage from a cyst
- Injury to adipocytes results in a chronic focus of granulomatous inflammation or an area that evolves into a lipid cyst with circumferential egg-shell calcification
- Mammographic findings include no lesion, a water density lesion, a mixed density lesion or a cyst with egg-shell calcification
- Ultrasound findings include focal fat oedema, an irregular hypoechoic area with no benign and no malignant features (Fig. 18.11), complex cysts with or without septations or a cyst with egg-shell calcification.

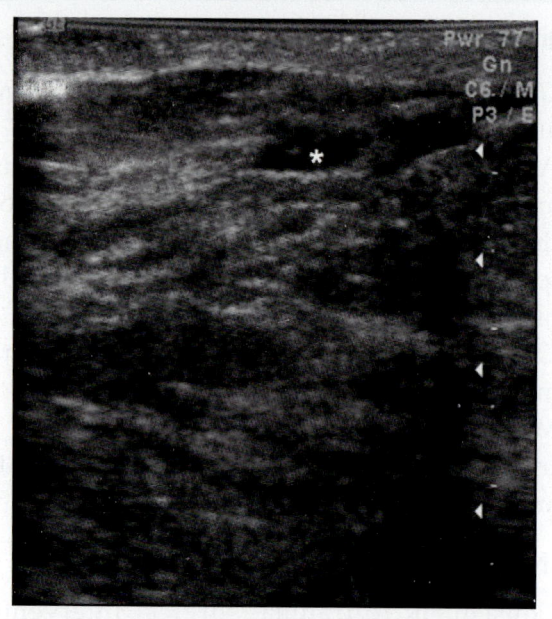

Fig. 18.11: The usual ultrasound findings in fat necrosis is a hypoechoic area with no benign and no malignant features

Mondor's Disease

- Refers to superficial venous thrombosis
- Presents as a non-compressible vascular channel which has internal echoes and may be variably dilated
- Tracing the lesion along its axis is diagnostic.

Hemangiomas and Venous Malformations

- Capillary hemangiomas present as echogenic solid nodules

COMPLEX CYSTIC LESIONS 159

- Cavernous hemangiomas and venous hemangiomas may present as variably echoic focal lesions with anechoic spaces that demonstrate slow flow vascular signals.

Lymphangiomas

- Usually axillary in location
- Consist of a cluster of simple cysts
- Echogenecity is consequent to the size of cysts, the smaller, more numerous and closer, the more solid appearing the lesions
- Lesions are very compressible.

Intraductal Papillomas

- These are discussed in Chapter 12.

Chapter 19

The Male Breast

- Conditions of the male breast are usually gynaecomastia, a palpable abnormality or a nipple discharge.
- Since the male breast is usually small and male breast cancer is usually non-calcific ultrasound is as good as mammography for assessment.
- Routine mammographic screening is not recommended in the male.
- Benign lobular processes such as fibrocystic change and adenosis are rare in males as lobules are poorly developed.
- Pathologic lesions are histologically and sonographically similar to those in females.
- Breast cancer in the male is usually seen in a breast with gynaecomastia and a history of trauma is common for reasons that are not clear.
- Lymph nodes in the axilla are common at the time of presentation.
- Metastases in the breast are usually from the prostate.

Section 4

Post-treatment Evaluation

Chapter 20

The Augmented Breast

Ultrasound evaluation in patients with breast implants involves assessing not only the implant but normal breast tissue as well.

Compression and harmonic imaging greatly improve visualisation at depth and minimise near field reverberation artefacts.

The normal implant has a host of different morphologies depending on the structure of the shell and the contents. The shell may be smooth or textured. Smooth membranes are thinner and more echogenic. Textured shells are less sharply delineated, thicker and less echogenic. Shell delineation is enhanced by employing higher frequencies. Saline can be differentiated from silicone because sound travels slower through silicone. The chest wall behind a silicone implant, therefore, appears deeper than it is. The echotexture of saline and silicone is similar. Over 200 types of implants exist and most women do not know which commercial type they have in place.

Long-term complications (Fig. 20.1) of implants can be well assessed with ultrasound. These include:
- Rupture
- Capsular contracture
- Haematomas, Seromas or Infection
- Migration
- Herniation
- Calcification
- Autoimmune Human Adjuvant Disease
- Carcinogenesis.

THE AUGMENTED BREAST 167

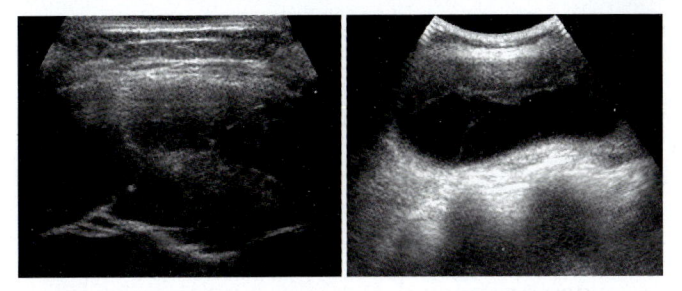

Fig. 20.1: Breast implant with thin and thick internal septation and low level increased internal echoes indicating shrinkage of the implant.

Rupture

- May be intracapsular or extracapsular
- Varies from a small tear to complete collapse
- Usually a clinical diagnosis
- The role of ultrasound (Fig. 20.1) is to identify granulomas or coincidental masses that may need a sampling or excision at the time of explantation.

Capsular Contracture

- Microleaks from all implants soon after placement results in a host foreign body reaction with formation of a fibrous capsule; this may become an exaggerated host response and result in implant capsular contracture
- Eccentric or excessive capsular thickening (more than 1.5 mm) can distort the implant.

Herniation

- Implant herniation through fractures in the capsule resulting in a clinical bulging
- This can be assessed by ultrasound and only rarely with mammography.

Calcification

- This is not unusual and of no clinical consequence
- May be focal or diffuse
- Can masquerade as a morphologically malignant lesion if explantation is carried out without capsulectomy.

Seromas, Hematomas and Cancers

- These appear as they do in patients without implants.

INDEX

A

Aberrations of normal development and involution 80
ACR BIRADS categorisation 66
Anechoic tissues 63
Assessing the breast lump 91
  ultrasound diagnoses 93
Augmented breast 165
Axillary lymph nodes 44

B

Benign and malignant lesions 77
Benign lobular processes 162
Benign lobulations 101
Breast 34
  accessory breast tissue 35
  branch ducts 35
  larger ducts 35
  lobes 35
  lobules 35
  lymphatic drainage 43
  nipple 34
  normal breast 39
  schematic representation of breast tissue 38
  subareolar duct 35
  tail 34
  zones 38
    mammary zone 38
    retromammary zone 39
    subcutaneous zone 38
Breast cysts 140
Breast implants 166
  long-term complications 166
    autoimmune human adjuvant disease 166
    calcification 166, 168
    capsular contracture 166, 167
    carcinogenesis 166
    haematomas 166
    herniation 166, 168
    migration 166
    rupture 166, 167
    seromas or infection 166
Breast lesions 132
  cystosarcoma phyllodes 136
  ductal hyperplasia 132
  hyperplasia 132
  juvenile papillomatosis 134
  phyllodes tumour 135
  radial scars and sclerosing papillomatosis 135
Breast lesions 60
  hyperechoic 60
  hypoechoic 60
  isoechoic 60
Breast ultrasound 3
  history 3
Breast ultrasound (BUS) 4
  indications 4
Breast ultrasound techniques 5
  aim 5

C

Calcification 15
Central ducts 48
Circumscribed cancers 97
Circumscribed lesions 100
Circumscribed tumours 100
Complex cystic lesions 145
    fat necrosis 157
    galactoceles 146
    haematomas 157
    hemangiomas and venous
        malformations 158
    intraductal papillomas 159
    lactational mastitis and
        abscesses 149
    lymphangiomas 159
    Mondor's disease 158
    non-puerperal mastitis and
        abscesses 152
    seromas and lymphoceles 156
    tubercular mastitis 154
Complex cysts 143
Compression and harmonic
    imaging 166
Cooper's ligaments 48, 150
Cystic lesions 139

D

Desmoplasia 96
Desmoplastic lesions 97
Doppler signals 88
Duct ectasia 87

E

Echogenecity 59

G

Galactography 90
11-Gauge directional vacuum-
assisted biopsy 86
Gynaecomastia 162

H

Haemorrhagic cyst 40
Histological basis of image
    morphology 86
Hormone replacement therapy 41
Hyperechoic tissues 64
Hypoechoic lesion 99
Hypoechoic tissues 63

I

Internal echoes 143
Interventional procedures 90
Isoechoic tissues 63

L

Labelled cystosarcoma phyllodes
    135
Lactiferous sinus 37
Lesion location 55
    five component code 56

M

Magnesium 48
Male breast 162
Malignant lesions 105
Mammogram 92
Mammographic BIRADS
    categorisation 66
Mammographic practice 96
Mammography 96

Mammosound 73
Microcalcifications 60
Microlobulated nodules 89
Microlobulations 101, 121
Movement of debris 48

N

Needles 60
Nipple discharge 85
   causes 86
      carcinoma 86
      duct ectasia 86
      fibrocystic change 86
      hyperplasias 86
      hyperprolactinaemia 86
      large duct papillomas 86
Non-calcific ultrasound 162

O

Oestrogen 41

P

Photoediting software 24
Premalignant diagnoses 131
Pulsed radiofrequency devices 75
Punctate calcification 142

R

Radial orientation 37
Real time 2D grey scale 20
Recent technical developments 19
   automated tissue
      optimisation 24
   colour Doppler 28
   harmonic imaging 20
      limitations of harmonic
         imaging 22
   power Doppler 28
   spatial compounding 24
      advantages 24
      limitations 26
   spectral Doppler 28
   virtual convex imaging and
extended field of view 26

S

Scanning planes 52
Scanning techniques 51
   compression 54
   fremitus 54
   mammographic correlation 53
   scan speeds 53
   simultaneous palpation and
      scanning 52
   split screen image 53
Schwann's cell 129
Silicone implant 166
Simple cyst 140
   benign 140
   cluster 141
Simple filtration 20
Solid breast lesions 107
Solid lesions 115
   diabetic mastopathy 126
   fibroadenomas 116
   fibrocystic changes and benign
      proliferative disorders
      130
   focal fibrosis 125
   granular cell tumours 129
   hamartomas 123
   hemangiomas 130

intramammary lymph
nodes 122
lipomas 124
pseudoangiomatous stromal
hyperplasia 128
tubular adenomas/lactating
adenomas 120
Solid lesions 95
benign versus malignant 95
Sonoanatomy 68
Specific features of some
malignant lesions 111
breast carcinomas 111
colloid carcinomas 112
ductal carcinoma in situ 111
infiltrating duct carcinomas
111
intracystic papillary
carcinomas 112
invasive lobular carcinoma 112
lobular carcinoma in situ 111
medullary carcinomas 112
non-Hodgkin's lymphoma 113
small tubular carcinomas 112
Spiculated tumours 101
Staphylococcus aureus 149
Sub-areolar nipple complex 48

T

Technical specifications 10
Terminal ductolobular units
(TDLUs) 39
Time-gain curve (TGC) 62
flat TGC 62
steep TGC 62

Transducer 10
transducer frequency and
stand-offs 10
resolution 13
axial 16
contrast 16
lateral 13
spatial 13
Transducer considerations 52

U

Ultrasound beam 47
Ultrasound BIRADS
categorisation 66
BIRADS 1 68
BIRADS 2 68
BIRADS 3 68
BIRADS 4 and 5 68
Ultrasound guided needle
procedures 72
abscess drainage 74
biopsies 74
cyst aspiration 74
ductography 74
general steps 72
radiofrequency ablation 75
Ultrasound morphology 87

X

X-ray galactography 86
X-ray mammography 4